NEW DAD HACKS

A Modern 4 Step Pregnancy
Guide for First Time Dads, Use
These Shortcuts to Help You
Feel Prepared and Transition Into
Fatherhood

By William Harding

contained within this document, including, but not limited to, —
errors, omissions, or inaccuracies.

Just For you!

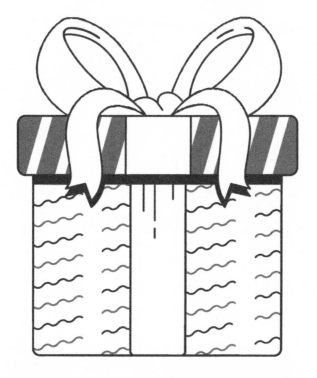

A FREE GIFT TO OUR READERS

10 Step **Action** plan that you can download now. Feel confident and prepared for your new born right now!

http://williamhardingauthor.com/

Table of Contents

Introduction

The thing that shocked me most about becoming a dad the first time was the feeling of helplessness. No one sent me the memo. Somehow, I figured that when I heard that baby cry in the delivery room, the challenge of the previous nine months was over. I expected it would be the time I could sigh in relief. All the stuff I hadn't been expecting over the last six months of life-changing events — mostly explored through my partner's emotions, cravings — would revert like clearing the cache on my browser. The rest would take care of itself. Or at least my wife would take care of it until the kid could talk and play catch.

Part of the reason I had no idea what to expect was the fact that birthing classes mostly covered everything up to the moment of birth. They covered a lot of practical things but ended up being all about what we would experience during the pregnancy from mom's point of view, packing a hospital bag, and preparing for the main event that was like a vacation at your in-laws. There were no dad-only nights where you got the lowdown on hormonal changes and the importance of shopping for a whole new wardrobe for months on end. The fact that the shape of my partner became alien was the easiest part to deal with because a lot of other things changed. Finances had already started to change, and many things shifted gradually and dramatically toward a baby orientation that I tried to limp through while supporting my spouse, who seemed to innately know how everything was supposed to work. Her confidence and knowledge didn't exactly rub off.

I learned to strap disposable diapers on a dummy; it wasn't very hard; nothing was moving. I even studied up on the finer points of fitting cloth diapers. It was an art similar to that of folding a flag. I passed the test in class, got my boy scout badge, and graduated. When I jabbed the dummy with the giant safety pin, it didn't scream or bleed or make me feel guilty. The dummy wasn't crying and peeing and writhing and pooing again just when I got the diaper off or just when I got it back on. The actual event of changing a diaper on something live was like trying to put a wetsuit on an otter that would rather be swimming. In reality, it was sometimes hard to figure out what I was supposed to clean first because the octopus of unpredictability had been released. Not only did I not know what to clean, but I didn't know what I was supposed to clean it with.

The first few times when my wife handed me the baby, I held it out at arm's length with two hands and stared at it like I was looking for a place to set down. It was like a gifted garden gnome that some friends gave me, and they were coming over for a backyard barbecue, and I didn't want them to feel bad that I ignored their generosity. As I held it out, it invariably started crying and had to be rescued from my grip, which was too hot, too cold, or too much like broken glass. Later I came to find that when you learned to warm up to the baby, it learned to warm up to you. Simple things don't always come to mind first when internally you are panicking about what you are doing wrong. Worse, you are the mythical man who won't stop to ask directions — sometimes even rejecting perfect instructions from a GPS. Often what you don't know, your spouse might, and surely someone else on the planet already does. It's a baby, something the earth's population says was done at least billions of times before.

I didn't have the tools, breasts, or whatever makes mothers, mothers, and dads like animated cacti. My wife would hand it to me, and it was like flipping a switch to tell it to cry. It was like the experience was some life lesson it had to go through to learn about life's cruelties, and I was its personal dungeon of pain. The baby had to learn that, during life, comfort was going to go to some other part of the house now and again, and you have to accept you needed to wait for solace to return.

Most of the real problem ended up being the lack of information. No one walked up to me after I handed out the cigars, pulled me aside, and said, "Hey, William, I've got some news for you." That sage advice I might expect from a buddy about what I got myself into wasn't on its way in person, in a text, or email. It was easy to see that friends I used to hang out with after work on Fridays started to become extinct when they got the news they were about to have a kid. They just dropped off the map not long after that, and I didn't see them anymore. I didn't realize they found out they had a family and their responsibilities changed, and I certainly hadn't had my opportunity to know what that entailed. They were a deafening silence dealing with their own adjustments hung up on the exact communal phrase: "this isn't going the way I expected." Their new cloak of stressors was something they signed up for and might even have been excited about. Like me, the only way they could take on the weight without collapsing was to double-up on the support of their partner and try to become a student of the changes that were going on.

Realistically, I knew there were sacrifices I was going to have to make in return for the gift of bringing a child into our lives. I just didn't know which sacrifices they were or how to handle them. If you take a look around, it is evident that people live through the experience of having children all the time, and some of them are men. I had no idea about the more subtle ways to test my ability to maintain my emotional maturity and composure. I was forced to absorb some duties that I certainly never mastered before I was married and that my spouse assumed the bulk of during the early part of our relationship. Looking from a distance, nothing suggested it was time to start a marathon study for an exam on becoming an adult.

Luckily we were expecting to be expecting. We were trying. Even that was a little strange as romance took on a whole different dimension when it was guided by a thermometer that told my partner when she was "ready." I've tried to do that, and it doesn't work very well. It was as if a third wheel entered into the relationship and some of what was fun (it still was) became an obligation driven by an inanimate object. That was just the beginning of the changes we needed to experience as a couple accepting our entrance into this new phase of our relationship.

For those men who happen to encounter this experience by surprise, that is a whole other level of revelation. Some people call it shock and awe. That's usually used in war and a precursor to PTSD. You'll be shocked at the news, wondering if you heard the right thing, and then everything will go a bit numb and dark around the edges as you discover tunnel vision. If your significant other just handed you a copy of this book and she didn't tell you the results of the second pregnancy test she took, you can only guess why she left it in your hands. Surprise!

Whether the news of fatherhood was planned or a total surprise, your experiences, as the situation slowly evolves, doesn't have to be shock and awe; you CAN manage the changes. My second child was way easier than the first, which is pretty much the rule for everything. The difference was I'd already been through the gauntlet. I found out I still had a few things to learn, but it was far less daunting because of the experience I already had. I would have been better at it if I had started with the second one. Regretfully, this isn't a box of chocolates. You've got to handle the arrival of your children in order—no magic pills or do-overs. Beyond the news of your successful conception and cigars and birthing classes, you need a short course for dads like you. This book is your guide to joining the Dad's Club. The journey starts by just putting one foot in front of the other.

The long, eventful, and rewarding journey you are about to enter is the life of being a father. It all becomes a lot easier when you know the things you need to know because the unexpected surprises won't be there. You can engage in and enjoy the process of learning about the new little adornment to life's experience. This could be your path to experience a whole new type of joy, and, when approached with some savvy, you can experience greater intimacy in your partnership as you strengthen bonds and responsibilities that ultimately tie you together. This book is your map, a guide to help inform you about what may be in store for your future as a new dad; you will be far better equipped for this journey with a few hours of committed reading.

> **"Every dad, if he takes time out of his busy life to reflect upon his fatherhood, can learn ways to become an even better dad." — Jack Baker**

My name is William, and I will be your tour guide. I am the veteran of participating in the experience of bringing no fewer than three new lives into this world. While I was innocent, stressed, and occasionally overwhelmed during the first expedition, I eventually made the adjustments and absorbed my new roles as a father and spouse. Not only that, I wasn't swallowed by the experience of becoming a father as I first felt was going to be the case. I was lucky enough to have a good job that gave me some freedoms that helped cushion the changes I was bound to go through, but even without that, I know now that everything would still have been OK. It would have been even better if I'd had worked harder to gain more insight. But that I was able to manage it walking through the experience and being blindsided at every turn means that you have an advantage that I didn't.

Part of the reason for digging in to write this book is my experience. I know it doesn't have to be a long, strange trip to work through the evolution of your immediate family. Looking back at my experience gave me confidence in approaching the next two wonderful gifts in the expansion of our clan from a nucleus of just two into the group of five I now adore and enjoy. When I found my good friend happily handing out cigars, I stepped up. After he'd made that initial announcement of expecting an addition to his family, I did what I'd hoped someone would have done for me. I put my arm over his shoulder and said, "Hey, Alex, I got some news for you." I offered some encouragement, but more than that, I offered to be there to coach him, answer his questions and talk about the stuff he was going to go through. I often beat him to the punch and sent him a message or three about where his life was heading when I recognized frustration or another milestone.

Seeing his response and feeling like I'd helped him, I was quicker to offer my support to my next buddy, who was setting out his wagon train to the wild west. Eventually, I was inspired to start an informal group for men, specifically for guys who no longer met up on Fridays after work because they were expecting their first. The goal was to help men seek some comradery, share experiences, and learn about what to expect as they traveled into unknown territory. More, it helped bring back some friends that had fallen into pregnancy and parenthood but neglected their own emotional well-being.

It has been seven years since my journey into this phase of my life began. The joy of that experience and the pleasure I took in helping others weather the storm of surprises brought me here to a point where I hope to help even more newcomers to the world of fatherhood. I know I've gotten better at being a husband and a father, and I am sure that I can help others learn from my struggles and successes in the challenges ahead. Like achieving success in your career, studies, or on the playing field, it will take some effort, but the results will be worth it. Confidence will give you more space to enjoy the experience and let that attitude of joy bleed into everything else you do while making you an enthusiastic participant instead of a casualty.

Let's get started on this new adventure. It may be a little like sky diving the first time, but we're jumping out of the plane in tandem, and I've checked the equipment and got you covered. It is a thrill I guarantee you will live through, and perhaps you'll reach out and pay it forward.

Parenting and Partnering Power

"Parenting and Partnering Power" are short focus sections at the end of every chapter. They are here to help guide you by emphasizing essential points and tell you what you should be doing to help yourself become a super-dad. Read every one of these and set yourself into action to get the most from the book.

The first task to activate your parenting power is to dedicate some time every day to get this book read from cover to cover. If you can only set aside 20 minutes a day, you will get it done in about a week (about 200 words per minute). Don't just breeze through to get it done. Concentrate on what you are reading and let it sink in. If you are pretty sure you glazed over something, don't cheat yourself; make a point to reread the sections the next day instead of moving on just to get through it. Dedication to reading is a little investment in the rest of your life, and it will be worth it.

Chapter One:

Yikes! You're Going To Be a Father

You just heard that you are going to be a father. No matter where the news came from, whether you've been looking forward to hearing those words or becoming a dad is a total surprise; you will likely be experiencing a wave of emotions, like a guy walking into the surf at the seaside. Whether you step into the violent uncertainty of ocean breakers or gentle lapping wavelets in a lagoon depends on the beach. Still, either way, there are rip tides and scary things under the water that were just waiting for you to get your feet wet.

One good piece of advice to follow, no matter how the surf is behaving, don't go swimming alone!

When you find out your partner is pregnant, you will have mixed emotions that can run to extremes. After all, it will be the day you realize something has definitively changed, and it will significantly affect your life from this point forward. This point in your life is a little like stepping off the landing at a bungee jump. The initial reaction might be fear, joy, surprise, trepidation — I'm not going to try and limit what you feel. Unless you've got narcolepsy, one thing you won't do is sleep through that initial moment of "what do I do now?"

The importance of empathy can not be stressed enough. The pregnancy is not something she is solely responsible for. It is something that you are both about to go through. Being empathetic and caring starts from the moment, you learn about the pregnancy. That moment when you hear the news, you might be tempted to be a bonehead and blurt out something that immediately comes to mind.

* "Are you serious?"
* "How did that happen?"
* "I thought you were on birth control."
* "Is it mine?"

This is not recommended as a starting point. If you've already started with the bonehead move, time to step back, regroup and grovel. You had a moment of pessimism that passed, and now you can beg forgiveness to clear the air and restore the regularly scheduled tempest. Depending on the situation, she may not have expected you to be overjoyed, but she will expect you to be part of her team. That may not take much more than a smile and saying, "I love you."

Your Partner, Your Strength

Something that often seems to calm a restless soul is finding someone who shares your perspective. The wonderful thing about pregnancy is that you and your partner are immersed in the reality of the pregnancy and tethered to it simultaneously. You are both in the same boat (yes, another analogy relating to water). If she doesn't make the first move to start talking about how she feels or asking you how you are with the news, there is nothing that's stopping you from sharing how you feel or trying to draw her out. Someone has to take up the oar, start the motor, or lift the sail. The ship has to get underway. Someone has to steer the boat. The crew has to work together. Some of the responsibility will be assumed automatically, but communication is imperative as you sail away into open waters. A lot can go wrong if the team is not in harmony with each other and the motion of the sea.

You may be used to taking the lead in many parts of your partnership, but on this excursion, you don't have to be the captain. A woman will probably be more prepared for what's on the horizon. Your partner will have paid more attention to her friends who are having children. She will likely have gained a sense of nurturing and nesting as a part of her nature and experience. You, on the other hand, are like a man sent out to buy tampons. You may be looking at pregnancy like a bunch of shelves loaded with boxes of brands, things you have no experience with. If you are like me, rather than asking your partner for direction, you'll wait to watch a few women make their selections while pretending to be looking at something elsewhere in the aisle. Then you can use the knowledge gained as a voyeur to come to a conclusion.

You may be sad to hear that the aforementioned male response to never ask for directions is the wrong response to your partner's superior knowledge of a subject. This new phase of your relationship is an opportunity to learn more about one another. One thing she will appreciate is that you show interest in what is happening. She may even understand that you seem to respect her knowledge of what it is like to be a woman and how she feels about the experience of pregnancy and childbirth. You may have goofed up and brought home the wrong box of tampons, but pregnancy is a much bigger thing that you aren't just going back to the store to exchange. It is OK not to know what being a pregnant woman is like, especially if you are a man. Asking your most intimate friend about it is sharing and bonding that can lead to sometimes alien things like respect and understanding.

At the same time, when you flounder in your ignorance and timidly approach her to share her wisdom, don't think she'll be all cool, calm, and collected. There are reasons for that, including raging hormones and her insecurities and uncertainty. This is something that she will physically experience for the first time, and that experience is far more immediate. You will both be stressed — be that from different perspectives. Any time of stress is a time where people are more apt to expose themselves emotionally, and sometimes being calm and rational is not the first step. Some might consider emotional exposure to ultimately be what a relationship is all about. One of the best things you can do is work at trying to explore the phenomenon together.

Before you start out with the map held upside-down, stress is not a bad thing. It is simply arousal that makes you more aware and alert to your surroundings. It is something you can use to your advantage to be more mindful and live in the moment. You are more likely to accept and achieve in a stressful situation if you take ownership of it rather than letting it run over you. In this case, taking ownership is sharing the experience with your partner. Working together through planning stages, sharing fears, joys, ideas, and responsibilities can help make your bond stronger. That will help throughout the pregnancy and into the years of learning the ropes of dealing with the baby, toddler, child, and teen as the wonder you created emerges and matures. It is a time to build strength and stability with headlights looking into the future.

The Physical Burden

In most ways, the physical burden of the pregnancy will be on the woman. She is carrying the living wonder in a symbiotic relationship as it grows inside her, and she is experiencing unfamiliar changes to her hormonal balance and physique. These changes can easily affect mood, endurance, and behaviors in ways that no one can predict. She may be alarmed and anxious about some of the changes, and it may be challenging for her to control her emotions. It is important to realize that while you may not be the one changing, you will experience the effects of the change either indirectly in her response to you because of how she feels or how the changes in your lifestyle affect you.

You may need to take up the slack when she is not feeling well and pitch in. Almost certainly, this is going to place additional demands on your resources such as time, energy, and sleep. This may mean skipping a card game, watching a sporting event, or a favorite TV show. It could mean waking a bit earlier to drop in a load of laundry or taking a shopping list out to the store after work. The effort will be easier to take on if you approach your partner with empathy and the situation with the understanding of the reward.

If you play your part true to the noble father-to-be, there is a good chance you may get pretty exhausted and even confounded by new responsibilities. These extra duties should never become a point of contention or resemble a contest of one-upmanship. You are trading the burden she has accepted by accepting some of your own to try to balance out the scale. While I was lucky enough to have some culinary background and could be called on in a pinch to cook, my household chores before my partner's pregnancy were generally delegated as "things that needed to be fixed." After pregnancy and my being steadfast in the idea that I didn't need any stinking directions, I didn't bother my partner with questions about doing laundry. That fear of admission led to parts of our white wardrobe shading pink. As it turns out, I needed lessons in folding clothes her way, which was more artful than my bachelor technique of piling things in a drawer. Back in the day, as long as the drawer would shut, the mission was accomplished.

Suppose you can bring yourself to always have the addition to your family as the light at the end of the tunnel, a muzzle on when a joke might be too campy, a mask of stoicism or empathy for those moments where the evil wants to erupt. In that case, you will dilute tension, quell turbulence, and avoid all earthquakes. Believe me, she is far more challenged than you are and at least equally stressed. Take the time to ask how she is doing and listen to what she is saying without flipping the channels on the TV. Your life is no longer only about you, and it isn't only about you and your partner. It is about engaging with the person you chose to live your life with to get through this experience with as much enjoyment as possible, as it leads to the next incredible stage of life together with a child.

The more you do pamper your partner, the more comfortable *you* will be and the more she will appreciate your effort. Bring her flowers, write a love note, and let her know you are excited about the future. You can't take her physical burden away from her, but you can help with the emotional burden by going just above and beyond at that moment where you think you did enough. Imagine if she just decided one day that carrying a baby was too much trouble. She's in no place to affect half measures, and neither are you.

You will have a lot of learning to do, and different stages of the pregnancy will require different levels of sainthood. If your mother-in-law is around, you might find you start to like her more as she jumps in to relieve you of some of the burdens and extra responsibilities around the house. A little praise sprinkled there might do quite a lot. We didn't live far from my partner's family, and I know they were helping out in ways I was oblivious to during the whole experience. I eventually learned more about that the second time around the carousel.

The infamous phrase "We are pregnant!" is not so much a statement of fact in the physical sense, but it is a declaration of your mutual commitment to creating a child as a couple. You won't be peeing umpteen extra times a day, and you won't get constipation and haveyour organs squish while you outgrow the shoe collection you bought as an adult, thinking that was the one size on you that could never change. But you can absorb some of the extra burdens and try to enjoy giving her downtime genuinely.

Show Her You Care by Educating Yourself

At some point, you will want to attend some birthing classes with your companion to learn more about your roles and some general idea of what you should expect. Don't ever get the idea that those classes prepare you for what's to come. They are something you do together, so it is an excellent show of commitment — just like accompanying her to doctor appointments. Showing her support in simple gestures lets her know you are in it together.

An even more impressive way to show your partner that you mean to be an active participant is to read about pregnancy. Instead of watching movies about the Darwin Awards for people who died in dumb ways or TikTok compilations that leave you in good humor but scratching your head, use that video time to man up by dedicating time to studying pregnancy and birth. This sacrifice of replacing something useless for something useful will serve a purpose when you mention a topic you'd like to know her opinion about and when you tell her what you learned about pregnancy.

Planning

In later chapters, we will learn what happens in four of the three trimesters. Yeah, that there are four trimesters is not a typo. Just because the baby is crying, that doesn't mean the game is over. The goal we are looking at here is to create a comprehensive plan for the expectant couple.

To be an effective partner in the pregnancy, it is wise to take on a planning role. It will force you to do some research into the realities of pregnancy and birth, learn about all the things you don't expect, and will help you feel reassured when the water breaks and it is showtime. Initiating the planning is not so much taking charge as building out your parental resume. You will take on your responsibilities in the role but share the planning with your partner. This also helps with communications and feeling out the expectations of each participant in the parental team. That makes sure the event is one you participate in like a partner and not like a wide-eyed lemur shocked into a frozen state by the rage of the machine.

Some of the most demanding aspects of planning for the long haul are budgeting and the birthing plan.

Budgeting. Beyond bathing in pee and potentially becoming intimate with parts of your partner's anatomy that even she will never see, discovering the actual cost of bringing a new member into the family can be the most surprising part of the pregnancy adventure. It is never too soon to start thinking about finances, even well before you think about having a baby. If you haven't thought about finances, the surprise, amazement, and wonder of learning that you have been involved in the creation of life can be supplanted by substantial sticker shock. Following this general mapping, budgeting includes considerations for:

* Wardrobe augmentation
* The baby room
* Baby care
* Time off work
* Medical costs

Some of these concerns may be offset by gifts from friends and family or work benefits but failing to consider any one of them may end up as part of a costly surprise. Failing to face the reality of which direction your life savings may be headed can only add to the stress of the situation and ultimately end in something resembling disaster. A financial disaster can be avoided by careful planning, putting aside money over time, and taking a good look at the benefits that your employer does or does not provide. Depending on where you live, various government benefits may also be available. New parents who are dedicated to making the most of enjoying their first baby can accomplish miraculous things even on such a short runway.

Wardrobe augmentation. Mama is going to outgrow practically everything during her pregnancy but her scarves. The rate of change won't be exactly constant, and the rate of growth due to the size of the fetus and genetics and eating habits of the mom will vary widely. Glamour is usually not the goal. Comfort, breathability, and practicality are more likely interests. Forbes says the average mom spends less than $1000 on maternity clothing. This relatively low number is expected because of the short-term length of wear, sharing between friends, and availability of low-cost maternity clothing options. Unless a mama plans to build her own army one soldier at a time, some garments may get no more than a few days of wear before they are retired. It is good to try and think of practical value rather than a radical fashion show.

The baby room. Even if there is a stand-alone room for the new arrival, a special place built just for the child can be advantageous. Nap times for the baby in a room behind her own door can be peaceful siestas with no interruption. Fitting the room with a crib and a separate changing table or chest of drawers does not have to cost a fortune. A practical matching grouping can be purchased anywhere between $200 to $1000 with a conservative budget. Be sure to check the safety ratings for any product that you buy using a platform that rates products publicly. It is never worth a few dollars saved to put your precious child at risk of harm. Keep in mind that these items may only be in use for a relatively short time and saving costs on the nursery to buy furniture to last the child through their teens is probably the wiser investment. A baby monitor is an inexpensive piece of added insurance against a baby's distress but can also be a soothing unobtrusive way to listen to precious sleeping breaths and cooing as children wake from a peaceful slumber. It makes up for the stresses of the inevitable crying.

Baby care. Baby care includes such things as formula, diapers, baby clothes, toys & teething, car seat, travel/diaper pack, stroller, carrier, nap seat, high chair. What you choose to get depends on what is important to you and your lifestyle, but all of this should be planned and purchased well before the trip to the hospital. Your choices matter. For example, reusable cloth diapers using a service and disposables can cost about the same price ($1000/year), but they have a different impact on the environment—research product ratings for anything you plan to buy with special attention to safety. Wood finishes on toys can be particularly deceptive as they may make things look dandy but could have long-term effects on a child's development. Chemicals and lead in a baby's diet are a no-no, and they will not discriminate as to what can and should go in their mouths. Keep all kitty litter out of reach of children, use safety devices on electrical sockets, and baby-gate everything that can't be child-proofed.

Time off work. Maternity and paternity leave are benefits some people get to enjoy depending on their employment and employer policies. For a fledgling parental duo, this one benefit may be a strategic reason for choosing one job over another when entering the child-rearing age. No doubt, parents with these benefits will want to take advantage of them. However, not everyone has this luxury, and when they do, the benefits vary widely between paid and unpaid time allowed. The key here is to be aware of any compensation that needs to be accounted for during any period that either or both parents will go without pay. It is good to plan for emergency time in case mom needs to take it lightly as her full-term approaches. Suppose the mother will not be returning to work for an extended period. In that case, the double whammy strikes where you have to account both for the lack of her financial contribution and the fact that baby raises household costs and lowers the limbo bar you have to squeeze under.

Medical costs. One of the unavoidable expenditures of pregnancy is medical costs. It could be argued that it starts with the pregnancy test and essentially never ends until the child is supporting him or herself. But the practical and immediate expenses of the nine months of pregnancy and subsequent birth are what is addressed here. There will be regular checkups with an obstetrician (the doctor specifically concerned with pregnancy and childbirth), tests (ultrasounds and laboratory tests), and the hospital bill, which can range widely between hospitals and methods of birth.

Without medical benefits, the cost of attended natural childbirth can be between $10,000 and $20,000. A C-section (where the child is extracted by an incision in the abdomen) can be up to $50,000. Things such as induction (artificially inducing labor) and epidurals (a medical procedure that taps anesthetic into an area of the spinal cord to numb the pain of the mother giving birth) cost more. Financially, it may be best to call a taxi after the water breaks and hope the birth occurs in transit. Due to the additional risks, that is not something you should pray for.

Ultimately, the cost of having a baby with traditional care if you have no benefits is somewhere around the same price as an inexpensive state university degree in the United States. If you have no insurance, had done no planning for the pregnancy, and it was unexpected, chances are you will need some type of social assistance or to take out loans that you will be paying off till right about when your 'baby' will be going off to college. Those are a lot of dollar signs to confront, and that is why it is a good idea to make plans before being surprised.

With benefits or other assistance, the costs drop dramatically, but studies suggest the average cost of childbirth, even with insurance, is about $5000. That can still be a significant sum to plan for, depending on your financial status. For other people, it may be the amount they spend monthly for online gaming fees. Now maybe the time to consider whether you could give up a non-essential expense to put toward your savings.

The point here is to make a financial plan. It may start by putting away a certain number of dollars from your weekly paycheck and should involve research into benefits and government support. List out everything you absolutely need, research the costs through your doctor and hospitals, and know what the total investment will be. At that point, you can make an informed decision as to how to cover the expense without loading up interminable debt.

Your Birthing Plan. While some experts consider 'budgeting' as part of the birthing plan, it seems to me to be too large in scope to squeeze in comfortably. The birthing plan is really just an outline of what you would like to think will happen during the birth and making some strategic notes about stuff you will not want to have to think of while they are happening. When the waters break, that is not the time to start looking for the keys or packing for the trip to the hospital. You want all of that done weeks and even months in advance.

The plan should contain a lot of boring-but-necessary stuff that will expedite everything. You don't necessarily need to include where the keys are, but you will want to be sure to develop a habit of hanging them on a hook by the door. This is one of several things

24

that are in the plan but remain unwritten. If you won't be driving and need or want to use a taxi, make sure they respond rapidly and include their phone number on the plan.

The written plan. Things you want to write into the plan include:

* Names and phone numbers of doctors and the hospital (and get these on speed dial on your phone).
* The schedule of doctors and appointment dates.
* The expected date of birth.
* Special concerns and considerations.

I doubt that I could have stated that last bullet point in a way that was any more vague. That is because the topic is vague. It will really have to do with the preferences of the mom for the birth environment and how the process should evolve. Listing preferences for music and available comfort foods may not be a bad idea, although that should be taken care of with the hospital bag (which we'll get to in a moment). More important things are preferences for epidural, natural childbirth, use of forceps, and birth location (at home, hospital, birthing pool, or taxi). A lot of this falls into the hands of the mother. Some may be decisions made by the couple as a team, such as baby names and circumcision preferences. This should pretty much include everything the mother can't contribute rationally while consumed by the pain of childbirth, and the father may not be conscious of doing having passed out from the things he did not expect to see. In other words, in an emergency where neither parent is capable, an attending nurse should be able to grab the page and locate everything she needs to know.

The unwritten plan. The unwritten daddy parts of the program include very practical things. No one will be worried about you because you are not carrying the package that needs to be delivered, but you have to be the tactical engineer.

* Know your job. If you are going to be in the room during the birth, be there and do what is expected of you. Make sure first that your partner wants you there for her support.
* Scope out the hospital. Take a hospital tour long before the time comes. Know where the admissions area is, where you can park long-term (all birthing episodes are not short), where the birthing rooms are (floor, desk, and arrangement), know where you can take breaks, locate something to eat, and where you might find a bathroom.
* Know direct and alternative routes to drive. Get to know the area and roads between your home and the hospital. If some freak backup happens, you do not want to get caught in it while rushing to the hospital (unless you are hoping for that taxi birth).
* Add your stuff to a hospital bag. Don't expect your partner to pack for you. Be ready to go at the first sign of contractions.

The Hospital Bag. It is best to pack a hospital bag and have them ready well ahead of the date the birth is expected. Even a 'normal' term can sometimes be shorter than expected. It is a good idea to have separate bags because the mom may need additional things. She won't necessarily be leaving the hospital right away. Separating the bags leads to less confusion when looking for things and allows each party of the duo to manage their own perceived needs.

You may want more or less than this, but here are some things to consider.

* Phone chargers
* Cash
* Entertainment
* Extension cord
* Change of clothes
* Toothbrush
* Deodorant
* Tissues or hand-wipes

Don't Neglect Yourself Entirely.

This process is going to be stressful and rewarding. You may actually come out the other side as a better person because you are forced to develop all sorts of empathetic tools. You will undoubtedly become more capable as a partner because you have to be responsive to your partner's needs and may have gained new abilities. You will be better prepared to be a dad because you have been building skills by just thinking about your family and the future.

While you have these improvements in yourself as a take-away, you'll still need to have some time out from the pressure of responsibilities. Be gentle in approaching this and also consider that you may be taking a break, but your significant other never gets one. Taking some time out to meet with your friends to go bowling or out for a run. Maybe you can break away for a sporting event. Whatever your interests and preferences are for taking a break, consider them well, keep them responsible, and make them short. If possible, take these breaks with some members of the daddy pool so you can multi-task. Sharing your experience with those in similar circumstances can provide insight and comfort. Do not go back home smelling of anything. Many pregnant women become highly sensitive to smell. Beer on your breath, wisps of the scent of a shared cigarette, and the stale odor of a bar will not be the best way to arrive home. Need I say that it is a bad time to visit a perfume shop, even if the gift is for her.

Be sure the time you will be spending out is covered by family or friends visiting with your partner. Do not leave her alone, especially later in the pregnancy. Allow your time of respite to be hers as well. A little time away from each other will help make invisible reparations even if things are going well.

Parenting and Partnering Power

This chapter presents many things to think about in the coming months, but empathy, communication, and budgeting should be things you engage first. These critical beginnings set the tone for a long time to come.

Get yourself a daddy notebook. In it, leave a page or two at the beginning to brainstorm ideas about what you need to include in your budgeting or just to doodle. Don't think of it as a chore, and make it your own. The more fun you have with it, the more you will use it.

The importance of writing out a budget and seeing how to meet it realistically can not be understated. Believe it or not, people do actually start saving for parenthood before they even know they are expecting. When you think it is time to start writing out budget considerations, give yourself ten pages or so to allow for expansion, changing your mind, and revisions. You want to leave room to revise in every section. You are not etching stone, so put the chisels aside. If you write with a pencil rather than a pen, your daddy notebook becomes a sort of whiteboard. With every section you create, consider making tabs with Post-its, so they are easy to find.

Make a section to collect things you need to discuss with your partner and use the pages to think of the best way to approach subjects that may be sensitive. Allow yourself to explore your ideas and feelings and make an effort to find ways to be communicative. If you are comfortable sharing the book, that's great, but you can also keep it as a journal, under lock and key.

Practice empathy and humility whenever you get the chance, and grade yourself on the response. If you reacted badly to something, write it down and think about how you could have done better. In baseball, hitters have good and bad at-bats. The best players learn from both. If you work on being sensitive to how your partner feels, you will get better at it, and your personal explorations will become a productivity tool for your relationship.

Chapter Two:

The 1st Trimester - Months 1 to 3+ (Weeks 0 to 14) of Pregnancy

Most people think of pregnancy as being nine months long. The gestation period for a baby is 40 weeks on average or about 280 days. That breaks not so neatly into trimesters of 14, 13, and 13 weeks each. The odd week has to fall somewhere. A good reason to think of the first trimester as the trimester with the flex week is that counting the start date of the pregnancy is not always very precise. Doctors usually mark the beginning of the pregnancy from the last date of menstruation. That isn't really very accurate in many ways, not the least of which is that conception will generally happen two weeks later.

When the page turns from "We're trying" to "We're expecting," it seems like that should come with a new attitude. Out of the gate, that attitude might be one of surprise and anticipation. There may be a spot on the roster for any feeling from the whole gamut of human emotion, fear, panic, giddiness, confusion, elation, joy, and the seemingly irrational syndrome called couvade (see the *What is Couvade?* Sidebar). Whatever the case, there is no prescription for your feelings, and there is no real prescription for her physical state.

Both of you will experience a change in one form or another, and working together to master the obstacle course is always a better choice than feeling like your partner should just buck up and deal with it. Life got more complicated with your willing participation, and it is a time to step up rather than flounder. It is actually quite likely that the challenges will do more to make you rise to the occasion and get better at being a husband and father.

What is Couvade?

Couvade is a sort of sympathetic state where men develop symptoms that are normal for a pregnant female to experience in reaction to their partner's pregnancy. This may include such things as backaches, cramps, dental conditions, nausea, and weight gain. All of this comes as an addition to your personal emotional roller-coaster, exhaustion, and consternation.

Some might argue it is purely psychological (psychosomatic), while others say it is due to actual physical changes that arise from extreme empathy and changes in the hormonal atmosphere of your environment (pheromones). In the latter case, chemicals that become plentiful in the air affect the natural balance of a man's constitution. That means the syndrome might be something like the McClintock effect, where women of child-bearing age sync menstrual cycles when they are in close proximity over a period of time.

Enough men (about 30% on average) experience the syndrome that is worthy as a subject of study. Even though I never had the experience of couvade myself, I'm still not one to poo-poo the possibility just because it didn't happen to me. It might be that I failed to be more emotionally in tune with my spouse or that I was not a good receptor for the other potential causes. If it were an emotional failing, that might be even worse than suffering the condition. At the time you would experience the condition is the same time that your spouse needs your emotional support and empathy the most. Because that is the case, try your best not to overplay your reactions.

To be a successful husband, partner, and father, you need a good understanding of the changes occurring with your partner, the baby, and how it is best for you to do what you can to meet the challenges posed by this partnership and be a champion.

Rising to the Challenge

The fragility of the early stages of pregnancy is nothing to ignore. It is a time when the fetus is most vulnerable, key developments are occurring, and interruption in the process could create complications. You have to be both the man of the house, sympathetic partner, and hall monitor to keep up with your end of the bargain. While you may already do manly things that require masculine strength, it is best to remain aware of what you can do to keep your partner rested and happy. Going out of your way to treat her a little like royalty will not go unnoticed. Special attention to small things, like not having to be told to take out the garbage while her sense of smell is overly keen, can keep her anxiety levels low and actually affect fetal development. Taking the helm on tasks you don't always engage in or initiate is part of assuming your new role.

If you didn't before, you now own all kinds of lifting, from grocery bags to dinner plates. If it has been since the early days of dating that you opened the car door for your partner, make it a practice again. Keep active, and you might just ward off some of the pounds you might put on when you become your partner's snack-mate. You get a double-whammy as the levels of stress increase, spiking your cortisol levels, which affects fat and carbohydrate metabolism. Don't do so much that you leap up every time she starts to speak, but remain conscious of those moments where you can relieve her of burdens. She will have enough to deal with during hormonal and other bodily changes, which only pile on top of her own concerns.

Be sympathetic to your partner by supporting her emotionally. If either of you smoked, now is a good time to quit. If you would like to share a bottle of wine with dinner, it is a good time for you to give that up when she does. It is also a time to start supporting each other's healthy habits. Getting outside together for a walk instead of one more hour on the couch watching Netflix can help set a precedent and nurture something the two of you and the child will benefit from.

The support you show her goes well beyond skipping a glass of wine. Certain foods are known to have a potentially higher risk factor in causing complications during pregnancy. Some of these foods are actually things that are ordinarily considered healthy when consumed outside of that 40-week window. If you had a sushi date night every week before the pregnancy, time to cut that out or be very selective in choosing only those delicacies that are fully cooked. Nothing resembling a raw egg, under-cooked meat, and cold cuts, or risky raw vegetables (e.g., bean sprouts) is allowed past the lips of the expectant mother. Cuts of large fish in any amount (e.g., tuna and swordfish) are not good choices because of the potential mercury content. Caffeine in moderation is acceptable but not recommended. Supplements of any sort should be brought to the attention of your doctor. Even vitamins can contain high doses of particular components, which are known to increase the risk of birth defects (e.g., vitamin A).

Potential dangers do not only lie within the mother's diet. While the baby can be pretty resilient in the protective cavity where it is encased, other environmental factors can play into the threats in a world it has not yet entered. Everything that comes in contact with the mother needs to be scrutinized because even seemingly harmless situations may bring about complications. If some of the mother's hobbies include woodworking, painting, and refinishing projects, fumes from the products she uses can be hazardous to the unborn, even in ventilated areas. Salves may sometimes have additives that can be absorbed through the skin. Favorite herbal teas may include ingredients that are not recommended during pregnancy for various reasons. Calming hot baths or saunas may raise body temperature to unsafe levels for the fetus. Anything that may cause jarring that tears the placenta, like car accidents, falls, or amusement park rides, are all things that should be avoided. For goodness sake, keep her hands out of the kitty litter and wash yours if you come into contact. Hair coloring and getting nails done is never as important as the health of the fetus. If she has allergic reactions that can only be traced to the bathroom, have an expert check for mold and mildew and take care of those infestations. The key here is to be cautious, sensible, and aware rather than afraid.

In all, the mother's body needs a higher level of nutrition during pregnancy, and the best way to achieve that is with healthy, nutrient-rich whole foods. That means this will not really be a pizza and Cheetos festival. Cravings are a thing, and there may likely be strange combinations of foods, and the pantry might get over-stocked with snackaroos of all sorts when mom has a hunger-driven binge-buy. It may be unlikely and possibly even cruel to keep a pregnant woman on an exceedingly strict diet (although that will sometimes be necessary for particular conditions), but an ounce of willpower may mean a lifetime of difference for a child. For best results, take cooking into your own hands, build menus that reflect her food preferences as they change, and err on the side of caution. You are being conscious of you and your significant other, but you are feeding the engine running on the peanut sprouting inside of her.

If you adopt a plan to rise to the challenge, it may be an opportunity not only to strengthen your partnership but to build a better, healthier lifestyle, embrace responsibilities, and work at the core of improving the prospects of your family before it even technically manifests in the cries of the birthing room.

Stress and the Pregnant Father

This subtitle isn't entirely accurate as you are not physically carrying the baby, but you are carrying a significant portion of the burden. Unless you are a zen master already, there are moments where stresses will forsake you. If you are feeling empathetic, present symptoms of couvade, and catch yourself in fits of anger or moodiness, you have likely come to a point where you should practice behavior modifications to help control your state of mind. If you don't do something early on, the effects could bleed over into your performance at work, affect your sleep patterns and pitch you into an avoidable downward spiral at home.

Don't get this wrong. As stated in the opening chapter, stress is a performance enhancer. It provides motivation to encourage taking action. If you go about this the right way, you will be learning skills that can help you cope with all types of stressful situations over the long haul. Things like retaining calm during your toddler's temper tantrums while out shopping will be easier to handle, you'll be more metered in your response, and ultimately you will be a better parent all-around.

There are many ways to practice the art of composure by taking simple measures. Saying "I need a drink" isn't one of them. The goal is to be mindful of your stress levels and build practices into your everyday life that make maintaining your cool second nature. When you practice and master techniques for keeping a cool head, you can free yourself from medications, become more cognizant and efficient, and simply brush away the demons before they can possess you. If you develop several tools, you should be able to practice it anywhere to quell everything from road rage to panic attacks. Some tools you might begin to practice with are:

* Breathing
* Meditation
* Self Hypnosis

Breathing. By far, the most practical and easiest way to gain control of heightened levels of stress is breathing. The best thing about it is that lungs are something you always have with you and the process of inhaling and exhaling is something you have to do anyway. You don't even have to take extra time for it.

Because you do it from the moment you are born, you'd think that everyone on earth would pretty much be an expert at breathing. Such is not at all the case. There are better and worse ways to breathe. In fact, if you go about it wrong, you actually enhance your propensity to become anxious. Short, shallow breathing is akin to hyperventilation, but they are not at all the same. The difference is that hyperventilation is quick, deep breathing. Shallow breathing deprives the respiratory system of oxygen. Either are poorly regulated respiration and cause a stressful imbalance in the blood oxygen level that the body will react to over time.

At its simplest, breathing methods range from just consciously focusing on the rhythm of your breathing to advanced techniques like Wim Hof's breathing methods or various breathing exercises (e.g., lookup 4-7-8, 7/11, and 4-4-4 breathing techniques). The timed methods just suggest the duration of inhaling, holding your breath, and exhaling. No matter which plans you choose to practice, practicing is the key to getting it right and having the method as your companion. Whatever you choose, do not push yourself with it to the point of discomfort. It is an exercise and not a weight-lifting regimen.

The common features of any breathing exercise are practicing breathing through your nose, breathing with your diaphragm rather than your rib cage, and controlling the pace of your breathing. Breathing with your mouth open bypasses an integral part of your breathing apparatus that helps filter allergens, dust, and germs. It helps to humidify the air as it passes through the nasal cavities and helps to avoid having a dry mouth or throat, which can lead to an enhanced risk of infections.

Breathing with the diaphragm helps you bring oxygen deep into the lungs. It helps in exhaling higher percentages of carbon dioxide while enhancing the efficient uptake of oxygen. People who take shallow breaths do not make the most of respiration, which can add to fatigue and other metabolic issues.

Make it a habit to breathe correctly and be mindful in times where you are not really able to do anything else. When sitting in traffic, in an elevator, in a line at a checkout, and any moment where you find yourself just waiting, take a deep breath or several. No one will be looking at you strangely for breathing. Eventually, you will do it automatically, and you will naturally develop a stronger sense of calm.

Meditation. Never thought you'd meditate? Time to give in and never say never. Meditation is probably one of the most well-known ways to achieve a sense of calm. Contrary to popular opinion, it is not necessarily spiritual, strange, or exotic. It doesn't require special tools or poses. At its best, it is absolutely the easiest thing that you can ever do for your well-being. Forget the incense and lotus position unless you like them. Meditation is a lot like a slightly more formal version of concentrating on your breathing. The most significant difference between meditation and breathing is that you will generally try to set aside a little time in the day specifically to practice meditation. Whether you choose to implement a mantra or simply breathe and allow your muscles to relax, daily practice of the ritual can yield benefits that last all day.

What you do during meditation is often said to be clearing your mind of thoughts. While that might be a goal for some, it should not be the only goal — if it is a goal at all. Thoughts will happen during meditation, just like dreams emerge during sleep. While meditating, you will try to let any thoughts leave as quickly as they emerged by not indulging them — especially if they are troubling. If you can learn to allow thoughts to pass, you can learn to let go of annoyances just as easily and stay on a more even keel.

Meditation, unlike breathing, is not automatic. It is something you practice and learn, and you will get better at it the longer you work at it. The totality of the subject is really the source for another book, but a lot of methods exist. Progressive relaxation (i.e., concentrating on specific muscle groups to release tension), guided meditation (i.e., following a guide's suggestions such as on a Youtube video), active meditation (i.e., moving in forms like Yoga, Qigong, or even walking), or visualization (i.e., picturing tranquil scenery or evoking calming emotions) are varied practices which may resonate with you. Try them all, pick what suits you best, and do yourself a favor and practice every day. Even if you only get in a few minutes, learning to control emotional bursts will help steady your response to triggers and curb the immediacy of your reactions.

Self-Hypnosis. It can be argued that there is really very little difference between meditation and self-hypnosis except that the reluctance factors differ. Some people don't like the idea of meditation because it appears too spiritual. Self-hypnosis gets branded by the misunderstanding that entering into a trance-like state allows other people to control your thoughts. In both cases, the preconceptions are untrue. While the consensus seems to be that self-hypnosis is different because you cross into a mind state that leaves you open to subliminal suggestions, those suggestions are meditations of your own. Self-hypnosis seeks an endpoint and a specific goal (e.g., reducing or eliminating bad habits), while meditation is geared toward absently experiencing the moment.

There is a lot of overlap between the two practices, and some people might prefer one over the other simply in name. In the end, the goal is to reach for an enhanced version of yourself so that you are a better you, a better partner, and a more effective guide in helping to nurture and raise your children. Take a look on Youtube for guided self-hypnosis sessions and try out the myriad of different styles which mimic the models of meditation.

Which Way Did My Friends Go?

There is nothing worse than a one-dimensional dad. Imagine growing up in the shadow of a cardboard cutout that really has no personality, interests, or passions. You'd just have a button to press to have money fall out of its pockets. The smile would be permanent and unwavering. It is a practical idea if you want your perfect family to be a Photoshopped wall-hanging.

The thing that a cardboard dad doesn't work with is emotional development. In a study that would be impossible to replicate with humans, psychologist Harry Harlow created a situation where rhesus monkeys were taken from their mothers within hours of birth. The mother was replaced with two surrogates, one that was a cloth-covered wire-frame that supplied nothing else and a wire-frame that was equipped to bottle feed. The study showed that the monkeys preferred the soft, comforting version of their mother to the one that simply provided food. Further studies in this area led to changes in how children were treated at orphanages, social services, and childcare.

The take-away point here is that if you are a cardboard cutout, your child will someday realize that there is little beyond the image. Instead of striving to be that perfect cardboard cutout, you will be most helpful and effective in raising your children if you actually have dimension in the form of interests, personality, and drive. This is where friends, hobbies, and adventure become inseparable from your value as a parent. Your genuine passion for a hobby, ability to interact with friends in a healthy way, and work on developing interests help nurture you. This, in turn, enables you to nurture your child. It also gives you and your partner a break from one another that probably leads to a more healthy appreciation of your relationship.

You can't just pause all aspects of your life because of pregnancy and hope to learn and grow as a person. Indeed, it is imperative to be heavily involved in and educated about the adventure your family has embarked on. Still, it is claustrophobic and deadening to make that the only source of stimulation in your life. You won't be good at turning off all your friendships and interests just to try to turn them back on when the time seems more convenient. You may have less time to dedicate, but don't let friends, hobbies, and interests fall off the map while you turn to cardboard.

The richer you allow your life experiences to be, the more you can share in your children's growth and their exploration as they move through life.

Immersing Yourself in Understanding Trimester #1

Knowing what the first third of the pregnancy holds in store for you, mother and fetus will make the whole experience of the events easier. I am absolutely sure that my participation the first time around was sub-par because I expected that what I needed to know would come to me. Instead, it likely was more of a case of: "Pfft. Nevermind. It takes longer to explain it." If you really want to be an asset in your partnership — and you should — learn about:

  * What is happening with the baby?
  * What's happening with your partner?
  * How can you best be of help?

What Is Happening with the Baby? In the first weeks of pregnancy, the baby is just starting to form, and by the end of the first month is still about the size of a grain of rice. While more features begin to emerge over the coming weeks, they are hardly recognizable. Even by the end of the second month, if you were to see the fetus, it would look more like some sort of prehistoric animal (or alien) than anything human. Four weeks more into the maturing miracle, the fetus is only about an inch long. It has managed to nurture more changes in your partner's physiology than its own.

Almost like the magic of a lump of clay becoming a beautiful creation in the hands of an artisan, the fetus looks far more human by the end of the trimester. The baby is still tiny and quite fragile. Even at that small size, the baby is essentially fully formed, although in miniature. The little fingers and toes begin to grow nails, and small movements begin in the extremities and jaw. While there is still not much size and mass, it is about three inches long and right about an ounce. For dads, let's say about the size of a strangely shaped baseball—the risk of any complications that have not already been identified drops significantly. Because the 14th week is recognized with the decrease in risk, it is often the milestone where couples choose to reveal the little miracle.

However, do not ignore that complications can still arise if you let your guard down. There is still no room for working with hazardous chemicals and cleaning products. Eating safely and paying attention to everything the mother encounters is critical to the fetus' further development.

What Is Happening to Your Partner? The sudden and grotesque emergence of hormones in the pregnant mother is nothing short of volcanic and chaotic. Even women who have proven throughout a relationship to be relatively stable troopers during the trials and tribulations of menstrual cycles may suddenly find their bane in the surge of blossoming motherhood. Picking a daisy may cause uncontrollable weeping. Swooning from nausea may lead to the inability to get out of bed with only the comfort of a vomit bowl and Saltines in close reach. Smells like the cologne she bought you for

Christmas may lead to hissing reminders to take a shower. Mind you, she picked the scent, and she now rages at it in a passion.

There will be no respite from the primordial response, and she can't take a pill to fix it without endangering the whole reason for the presence of the onslaught. The father might well be tempted to consider a vacation to a foreign land just for a short 14 weeks or so, but the truth is that this is when you may be needed the most. Getting screamed at in the birthing room is nothing compared to the potential tempest that threatens to cleave oceans in two and scatter the broken hulls of boats on the rocks. But the waves of turmoil can ease just as quickly to sad moments and calm. Changes in blood flow cause discomfort in the form of constipation and swelling of the breasts. It may be best to designate a particular bathroom off-limits to anyone but the mother if you have the luxury of more than one. The growing frequency of peeing increases in concert with nausea, and the whole makes having a b-line to the facilities all but essential.

What I described here is the worst-case scenario. Some women go through the first 14 weeks with barely any symptoms at all. Your spouse is experiencing a chemical cocktail as she has never had before. Just as patients respond differently to various medications, the result comes down to an individual's experience with their change. You might experience every bit of the horror, or barely any at all.

The question left to ask is: what is a father to do?

How Can You Best Be of Help? There is probably little that is more stressful than being helpless. In various animal studies in laboratory settings, animals are put into situations that seemingly can not be resolved. In these situations, the animals invariably surrender and accept fate. But this should not be the course of action for the educated and empowered modern male. Knowledge is your advantage, and sympathetic action is your key to success. You can't take the struggles from her, but you can be smart about the steps you take to ease her discomforts.

The first thing to do is to deal with your own problems. You are a better partner immediately if you are not bringing issues to her when she is under siege by her own body. While you want to commiserate with your partner in moments when she seems to be in the mood, do what you need to do to take care of your mental attitude. Do not express your suffering to her, and do not complain about how she is failing to handle her torments. Look back at the section on "Stress and the Pregnant Father" and start indulging your exploration into an embodiment of tranquility.

Notice her trends for her. She may not see that the cup of coffee she allows herself in the morning encourages the rise of magma at her core. Likewise, some activities, foods, or beverages might provide an umbrella of calm. If you have taken the advice from early on, keep notes to track her successes and outbursts and what seems to be a trigger. A resolution may come down to something simple and easy to control.

Consider yourself officially responsible for everything. When she feels up to it, she will possibly push you out of the way and take over certain things, especially close to the end of the first trimester. Just don't count on it. You should still never let her exertions be extreme, and anything involving more than hand soap is likely not something you want her getting involved in cleaning. Do not make her feel parasitic and lazy. Reassure her that you are doing what you can, and it is the least you can do to participate in your joint venture.

Romance like food can take on whole new directions. Cravings for either can emerge and wane. Try your very best to be supportive and flexible when satiating appetites or resist making ill-timed advances. Stay on call as the concierge and make your mission to serve. Both food and changes due to pregnancy will have effects on her physique. She may not feel attractive. Assure her that your attraction to her is not changing and maybe let on that you think she is beautiful.

Show some interest in the progression of the process. You might want to have a camera-ready (or at least your phone) to capture and share memories occurring during the pregnancy. Consider introducing a joint project like a baby book or maybe a modest web page to keep family and friends informed of the progress. Showing her that you care about this being something you have engaged in together may help quell her anxieties, doubts and shorten the swing in the pendulum of her moods.

When all else fails, it is time to listen and listen well. She won't always tell you what she is thinking exactly, and she may not be able to. You have to finally be the mind-reader she has always envisioned her prince charming would become, and you have no other part in the movie for now. She is handling the physical burden. She will get the attention. You will be more than a pack mule, but you might often feel like one. Beyond that tortured exterior, she is still your partner. She may not be mindful enough to have any regrets about outbursts and moodiness, and you should not expect her to. If you read this carefully enough, you know what's coming. With the right attitude, you might even enjoy it.

Come to terms with the fact that the hormonal changes in your partner are temporary. She will start shedding the masks of all her new personalities as the tide of hormones recedes. Assure her that you are aware but do it in very gentle ways. You are not in a good spot if in the middle of a tirade you blurt out, "I know that is the hormones speaking." As you turn your head away from her reception of the comment, something handy like a lamp may be headed toward your skull. You can probably depend on the cord being short enough to keep you from harm, but never underestimate the newborn athletic prowess of a woman in the throws of chemical change.

She may be terrified by the whole process and what she sees as an insurmountable mountain of trying to push a bowling ball through the eye of a needle. If you can clear the first 14 weeks without incident and lunge for the finish line, just know that there are only 26 weeks left to go. You will likely break your silence to friends by this point, and the marker for the second trimester can begin. Things might just get a little easier from here on out.

Parenting and Partnering Power

Now is your time to start building rituals. Some of these might only last through pregnancy, but all can be helpful, and some can improve the quality of life for your whole family for the long haul. You want to focus on being the hall monitor for anything that your partner does that she may forget could cause risk to the baby. You need to be gentle and empathetic about your approach. That doesn't mean setting up spy cams or flying drones around to follow every step she takes — unless it is a joke, and you know you won't scare her to death. Never scold your companion. That is a partner you are talking to, and you need to treat her like one.

Being alert and mindful goes hand-in-hand with tending to your own needs and building skills for controlling your emotions. Choose a method of dealing with stress and begin working with it immediately. It may help to start a section in your notebook to keep track of your exercise and make notes to yourself about what you are doing right. Learn from the mistakes, but don't be shy about noticing you improve.

Chapter Three:

The 2nd Trimester - Months 3 to 6 (Weeks 15 to 27) of Pregnancy

If the first trimester felt like anything less than running a marathon, consider yourself lucky. No matter how well prepared you thought you were (even if you read this book before it happened), you probably, on one occasion at least, found yourself experiencing a feeling akin to being blindfolded on a diving board off the side of a pirate ship. If you've come out the other side without anyone having to yell "Man overboard!" you are a champion. There is hope on the horizon. It may be time to take the blindfold off, taunt the sharks swimming in the waters below you, and step back on the ship. Not to promise anything because the unexpected can happen, and the effects of the first trimester can go extra innings. Still, something should be emerging; you should both be coming to terms with the 'routine' of being a couple that is expecting. That alone is a triumph.

You have probably developed some habits as to how to handle your new responsibilities in practice — which is the real reason reading alone doesn't make you prepared. If you've ever thought about going sky diving, you read about it to prepare, you took a class and read a book, and you knew everything about it, you wouldn't have to jump out of the plane. It is probably the one thing that root canal and having sex have in common: If you have never done it, all the preparation only gives you an idea of what to expect. When Dr Smiley says, "you are going to feel a little pinch," and the needle sliding into your gum-line seems to be the length of a samurai sword you have arrived.

The familiarity means you and your partner will both begin to experience less stress, whether or not the actual situation has improved. The period where you can both begin to enjoy the honeymoon period has arrived. If you opened up and announced the pregnancy at this juncture, you will be able to speak with people around you and share experiences and emotions you may have been hiding. You'll feel a little like you are emerging from a cocoon and experience the release of telling someone a secret you have been withholding — and that's because it is precisely what you were doing. By no means is this the end. You've only done three laps in this marathon, and there are six more to go. But just like a runner in a race, you've settled into a position in the field. You don't want to look behind, but you do want to look ahead to see where you will end up in this race and strategize as to how to make the best effort in greeting the finish line.

First things first. Take a look back at the things you didn't manage to accomplish in the first trimester and replicate them on to your to-do list for the second. It would help if you hadn't procrastinated, but you still have time to make up for it. Note down all the positive things you think you did and get ready to keep replicating those actions; focus on further developing the skills you see as benefiting your relationship and your family's future. You've got the battle scars, and should you have the luck to go through that experience again, it will indeed seem familiar, easier, and welcome.

We have an Announcement!

Before you rush out in traffic on your horse galloping through the streets yelling the news of the confirmed pregnancy to anyone who will listen, take a moment to plan. Passing the receptionist desk at work and flipping on the intercom to announce the new arrival is probably not the best way to go to work. The announcement that you and your partner are expecting should trickle down through the proper channels lest it runs upstream in a way that isn't natural.

Take every step to make sure those who will be hurt most by hearing second-hand news hear it first from you. Your boss goes before any of your buddies at work. Your parents go before a Facebook post. Having the sense to treat your allies with the respect they deserve will only help strengthen those bonds that you might just need as your experience continues and your need to rely on support expands.

The gesture of going boss-first drives home the implication that you respect that he/she will be affected by the potential shifts in your workload and days that need to be covered. It also speaks to the idea that you take your job very seriously. Asking for advice about how he/she prefers things to be handled also plays a political chip. Any time you ask someone for their advice, it creates an alliance.

Friends and family who already know when you take to social media will be likely to voice their support and help to be sure the word gets around to the corners of your social imprint. This will take some of the burden off you for alerting everyone you know, and you don't show up some months later to a party with a baby bump whose origin is suspicious to the host.

The announcement is another thrilling step, but good sense uses that to your advantage. Already your child is paying dividends.

Finances: Exploring Your Resources

If you have not yet taken the initiative to explore the potential benefits you can take advantage of, now is the time to delve in deep and search out information. Depending on where you live and your company policies, you may have a wide range of options for time off work (paid and not), coverage on medical expenses, and options for networking resources. This is only the tip of the iceberg.

You will want to visit the Human Resources department where you work to get the low-down on exactly what you are entitled to and when. You will treat everything as if it is predictable, even if it isn't. Unexpected situations can still occur, and having the knowledge about your options can give you the tools you need to make quick decisions about what to do should anything arise. If you look into it later, there may be other consequences, and for some benefits, it may just be too late.

While we have already touched on the topic of financial planning, the hectic atmosphere of the first trimester is not the best time to load up on that worrisome mountain beyond realizing the basic structure of [Baby] = [Costs Money]. Hopefully, that was enough to make you start planning ahead by regularly putting some money aside. This game has no "get out of baby costs FREE" card. Unless you happen to come from very privileged circumstances, this responsibility is one that you will have to bear. As the looming reality of medical costs creeps closer and the reality of 'baby on the horizon' has set in, you can more rationally deal with creating a solid plan. You will need to make an honest assessment of the money that is realistically available to you against what you will inevitably have to spend.

Resources to explore in-depth include the following. Do not be optimistic with any of these amounts, as that will only tend to lead to a shortfall.

Your current savings. This should include what you currently have saved as well as what you hope to accrue. By 'hope,' that is what you have already assessed to be an amount you can comfortably put away with every paycheck.

Employee benefits. Time allowed off may seem like a good thing, but it makes a huge difference if that time off is paid or not. Paternity leave will likely vary from maternity leave, so make sure you read the correct section in the Employee Handbook. If you have that benefit, it can help you make a substantial contribution to the transition from pregnancy to experiencing more of the child's earliest moments on the planet and support your partner in acclimating to taking care of the new addition to your family. Read the Employee Handbook and be sure to consult with Human Resources to confirm you got it right.

Insurance coverage. While the company you work for maybe provide insurance coverage, you want to treat what they accomplish separately. This will have to do specifically with medical expenses, which will be the most significant portion of the baby bill. Like employee benefits, insurance will vary depending on your plan and the company that the plan is managed through. Read your policy and be sure to give Customer Service at the insurance company a call to be sure you reached the correct conclusions and that you are not missing any benefits or inconspicuous requirements.

Social support. Under this category, you are looking at the potential for pledges by friends and family. Assigning an actual figure to this sort of support will be difficult. The friend who professes: "Don't worry about it, I'll be there if you need me" may have no real intention of following through or may not be able to when the time comes. You might want to keep track of that in a 'speculative' column of your formal financial assessment. The real value of social support is more likely to be donations. Unused baby carriages, cribs, changing tables, and other accessories can save you a lot of money. Especially if money is going to be tight when you reach the bottom line, there is no need to be overly proud about something that will only get short-term use.

Government programs. Depending on where you live, your income, financial situation, and other factors, your access to government programs and social support will vary. This is another situation where research, networking, and consultation can pay off. You will want to look up government information as well as consult with your obstetrician.

Credit lines. While getting into debt may not be your first choice, it may be one of the only ones if your current resources are not sufficient. Applying for a loan or taking out a second mortgage are ways to finance having a baby over time. If you are a first-time father and have not done much to build your credit score, having a child and taking out a loan might actually help your financial viability — so long as you can pay it back. You will have to keep up on payments, but the fiscal risk of a responsible parent is something that financial institutions look on as a positive. It could help position you for investing in the purchase of a home or upgrading if you already have one that will soon prove to be too small.

What is a less interesting option is financing the baby with credit cards. This kind of high-interest debt is something you want to keep to an absolute minimum (e.g., the occasional purchase of maternity clothing) to keep the accruing debt off the baby-costs ledger. Credit card rates can be as much as ten times the rate for a home-owners or personal loan. This kind of debt needs to be a temporary fix if you want to stay financially flexible.

What your budget should look like. Some people will never have had to budget, and that is probably because it ranks on the fun meter something like scrubbing your driveway with a toothbrush. Even thinking about a budget sent my wife into diatribes of denial, exclamations of the task's impossibility, and all manner of avoidance behaviors. The goal of a budget is more rudimentary than all-encompassing. Write down what you know, and not mystery expenditures. As with all seemingly impossible tasks, break it down into steps by working away at the easy things first.

If you and your partner have been together for any time at all, you will have an idea of the costs you have from month-to-month or week-to-week for rent/mortgage, grocery bills, car payments, insurance payments, electricity/utilities, internet, phone, current credit debts, etcetera. Just list out the known costs and add them up and compare that to your income. It may be painful to look at, but waiting will only make that pain more severe. The bottom line will probably affect your decision-making and will force you to be responsible. If there is an apparent shortfall, the goal has to become how to make the ledger balance.

If you can't just sit down and get it done, you may want to engage the services of a financial planner. The bad thing about that is that it will cost money. The good thing about that is that a good financial planner will be sure you have a solid plan, offer proper financial advice, and you won't have the opportunity to blame your partner for making big errors in the estimates.

Future Planning. Along with the pain of financial reality come other practical aspects of living as a family. Life insurance policies should be reviewed or considered. Plans for improving quality of life over the long-haul help you put together realistic plans for moving into a suitable residence, planning for your child to attend good schools, and even helping to launch them into their independence as a young adult. Starting a college fund is not out of the question. Beginning a savings account for your child to deposit any cash gifts can eventually turn into an account the child can manage for themselves to help make them responsible adults. It can be fun to envision what the future may hold for your child, and starting them early can help set them off on a path that espouses freedom and success.

The Mid-Pregnancy Scan

Sometimes known by the unfortunate name of "Anomaly Scan," mid-pregnancy is another milestone that you should prepare for but not fear. At this stage of the pregnancy, the fetus is large enough that the sonographer can detect fetal progress, including normal, healthy brain development, bones, limbs, features, and other organs. Scans also look at the development of the placenta and general health of the mother, and conditions that may affect the pregnancy having nothing to do with the child. It may be cause for further testing, bed rest, or other precautions.

While there is the possibility that you will get news that reveals something, this only happens 6% of the time globally. That 6% also does not mean whatever was revealed is automatically cause for concern. The percentage will vary depending on the country you live in and possibly even where you choose to vacation. For those without known risk factors in genetics, environment, or habits, the percentage is reduced by about 50%. It is good to go in with a positive attitude expecting a glowing report instead of working yourself into a hand-wringing frenzy. Becoming anxious releases hormones into the system and can create an imbalance of the body; what may begin as needless fretting could potentially trigger unwanted issues.

Scans are not perfect and will be dependent on the sonographer's experience and expertise to some extent. The scan will also not uncover every possible defect or condition, some of which will never be apparent until after birth, and some not until years later (e.g., colorblindness). It is also good to remember that everything considered a 'defect' is not necessarily serious, debilitating, or cause for concern. I was born with a preauricular pit which sounds ominous. It is just a tiny hole in front of the ear. My first daughter was born with the same condition, and when I saw it, I was actually a bit flattered that we shared an obvious common trait. But the key here is that fretting does nothing to change the outcome. The other side of the coin is that the scan will usually result in confirming that everything is progressing well. It is also possible to discover the sex of the baby. Know beforehand if you want that to be part of the discovery.

The scan itself is not invasive and will usually take around thirty minutes. There may be slight complications in getting a good view due to the positioning of the fetus and possibly the mother's own anatomy, but just hang in there, be patient and supportive of your partner, and reign in anxiety. If it wasn't obvious: be with your partner for the scan! It is incredible that some people choose not to attend this chapter in the miracle of birth and prefer not to be there to support their partner. The scan is not mandatory, it is not harmful to the mother or child, and the peace of mind it can offer is well worth going through. The results are available immediately, and some sonographers may give you a running account based on their style.

If anything is found during the scan, you will be informed, and any options you have will be explained. If a second technician either attends the scan or does a second review, it may just be the hospital's policy. The technician may have limited experience or may request a second opinion to ensure that all the results are correct.

Immersing Yourself in Understanding Trimester #2

Just like in the first trimester, there are certain things you can expect to be part of the baby's development, changes in your partner, how you fit into your role as an important part of the script, and maybe even what you've learned about yourself so far. We'll have a look specifically at what is going on, just like we did for the first trimester because when you know, you are a better partner.

* What is happening with the baby?
* What's happening with your partner?
* How can you best be of help?

What Is Happening with the Baby?

The baby has become recognizably human by the 14th week and is only going to start growing more rapidly. Starting at about 4 inches by week 15, the fetus will grow to about half an inch per week, getting up to about 9 inches by the end of the trimester with growth in bodily length accelerating.

During the first month of the trimester, the fetus begins to sexually mature, with males forming a prostate and females developing ovaries and what will mature into their life-long store of eggs of their own. Hair will grow along with a mucus-like substance (vernix caseosa) which helps to protect the skin in the aqueous environment where they are developing.

In the later months, the formation of hair extends to eyebrows, and other fine physical attributes such as taste buds mature. Your budding flower is essentially a miniature human in every way by the end of the trimester and only goes on to advance in these stages of development in the approaching trimester.

The "lump of clay" had made a significant advancement in taking final form. Remain diligent and alert to dangers in the environment. Try and be helpful with your partner's diet, which will continue to morph and flourish. Everything that passes her lips still plays a part in the development of the child.

What Is Happening to Your Partner?

Around week 13, many women begin to both experience the rambunctious effects of hormones as more tolerable and grow more accustomed to simply being pregnant. This trimester is the easiest part of the pregnancy for most women, and it will hopefully come as a welcome respite for you. There are, however, no guarantees. But you may see a smile more often, and the fierce swings in mood may become less volatile. At the very least, things should not get worse.

Don't let that suggestion make you think changes in her are finished. She may begin to experience other pregnancy symptoms, like joint aches and unusual flexibility. Her body is going to start seriously adjusting to what it needs to be able to do at birth and bust that bowling ball through the eye of that needle. Relaxing plays a major role at this point which helps relax smooth muscle tissue and foster growth of the placenta. While flexibility may initially seem like a benefit, too much of a good thing can lead to loose joints, injuries, and problems performing seemingly simple tasks like walking or standing up. It is nothing to be tremendously alarmed about but something to be aware of. If mom has difficulty, she may need to take it easy to avoid a serious fall and may need your help — at times more than she would like to admit. Remain understanding and resist the urge to dote.

Another biologically stimulating change your partner will experience is the enhanced presence of estrogen and progesterone. This will stimulate melanocytes' production, which affects the balance of melanin in her skin and can lead to a range of conditions. If she usually has clear skin and begins to get a bit blotchy, chances are she will not take to that kindly. She may develop a lina negra, or darkened line, vertically at her belly button. Her nipples will probably ripen to a darker shade, and moles or freckles may be affected by changes in color and possibly size or shape. It is important to note these things so they are not mistaken for something more serious. Cortisol and Human Placental Lactogen levels will fluctuate, affecting blood sugar levels, blood pressure, and metabolism. Unless anything seems to go haywire and she is experiencing persistent secondary symptoms, these changes should all be temporary and will not be dangerous to the mother or fetus. Simple changes in diet and exercise can control many resulting issues. She should consult her physician with any concerns.

Those are the common menu items. She may have any of these along with side-orders of indigestion, shortness of breath, congestion, constipation, gingivitis (or similar symptoms), fatigue, flatulence, swollen feet, blurred eyesight, and circulatory discomfort that may result in spider veins. Last but not at all least, there will begin to be physical evidence of what is growing inside. That baby bump and its swelling may be just what is creating some of the issues. As it expands in the limited space allowed, it starts to push organs out of the way and physically stress systems by putting pressure on them. In all, the smorgasbord of symptoms, annoyances, and issues will probably pale in comparison and nearly seem to be a relief when compared to troubling nausea and relative insanity of the first trimester. It may well be that simple systematic desensitization to the initial onslaught has made her a better warrior, stoic to the mere, trifling challenges that emerged. She has made it this far and, as such, has fought an admirable and inescapable battle. Let her know that you admire her effort.

How Can You Best Be of Help?

You, Prince Charming, will want to do all you can not lose the beautiful qualities you have nurtured in becoming a better human during the first trimester. You want to continue to nurture her, understand, help guide her to sound decisions for the sake of all, and hold fast to the righteous path. But now you have practise, you've grown as a person, and you are already a model that other newly expectant fathers can emulate.

Aren't you?

Here is an excellent time to take inventory of what you learned and did well, but hardly time to start awarding yourself prizes for excellence. People have to practice for a long time before they truly become good at something. Be aware of what you accomplished, know what worked and didn't, and learn from your mistakes.

Just like you needed to concentrate on maintaining friendships as a takeaway in the first trimester, don't let yourself get caught up in inactivity. At the outset of being a dad, your partner is going to have plenty of reasons to rest. She has to protect the asset she is carrying. She will be drained by doing nothing more than her body taking over to stoke her incubator. You might want to eat in sympathy so she won't feel bad for gulping down extra portions, but you don't have the same engine burning your fuel. You might try to involve your partner in walking or other exercises that benefit you both, but if you allow yourself to bloat out, you aren't going to get rid of a whole bunch of it in a birthing ordeal.

Stay mindful as to how to keep fit. Don't go punching elevator buttons when you can take the stairs. Don't try to find the closest parking space unless you are delivering precious cargo. If you are, act as a chauffeur and drop her at the door, then valet-park your family craft like it was a new sportscar that you don't want to be dinged on the first weekend you bought it. That means long and far away from the door so that you have to walk it. She'll still be checking in at the waiting room desk when you get there, and you'll have put in some extra steps. Put an app on your phone and try and set a goal for steps every day. Take a walk at lunch. Fill that step count, and if you see your own baby bump start to grow, up to your daily goal.

Contrary to most people's beliefs, walking can be just as beneficial as running. It is less stress on the body, easy to recover from, and has good cardio. Before this is all over, you are going to have still another leg of that marathon to run, and you will want to take it in stride while remaining healthy and prepared to take on fatherhood for the long haul. You are not too busy to get a little extra work in. You can clean while she rests, take the dog for a walk — anything that keeps your engine burning like your partners will be without her slightest effort.

Women will adjust to the changes in their bodies in different ways. Some may feel down about their metamorphosis. Here is where your reaction can make all the difference. If you communicate in a loving way that you sincerely enjoy the changes and stress the importance of her efforts and your joy in the idea of your growing family, that should come out well. Assuage her doubts about her appearance, be communicative, stress the positive, and you might find a benefit in growing your intimacy as a couple. Her response may take you by surprise, especially if the romantic side of your relationship took a vacation during the first trimester. You have to understand that it just isn't fun to make whoopie when you need to be sure the vomit bowl stays within reach.

You did great to get through that first trimester, and you will do fine in the second so long as you embraced your role, worked at being a great partner, and rewarded yourself for noticing the positive part of what you have done for yourself and your family. Don't lose sight of your friends and support network, keep making time for physical and mental well-being, and take joy in enhancing your relationship and interdependence. You are about to enter the third act of the play feeling like you've got the hang of this partnership thing. It may be a quiet celebration, but there is nothing better than taking on the challenge and improving yourself.

Parenting and Partnering Power

Homework for the dads to be right now includes taking inventory. If you made an effort with your notebook, birthing plan, and finances, you are going to be in good shape from the planning perspective. Continue your personal growth with diet, exercise, and stress training.

Professionals who use planners never write things down one time and never look at them again. Update your plans from time to time to incorporate what you learned or remembered you forgot. This means looking at your birthing plan and notebook to update everything that needs it. Change all plans that have evolved as they are bound to over time and as you gain experience.

It isn't a bad idea to do a monthly review because a lot of times, you will find yourself saying, "yeah, I wanted to add that." You might even pick a day of the month to do your reviews. It won't take you hours to do. Just a couple of minutes a month for review can keep you miles ahead in making your plans detailed and successful. Writing helps you think and discover, and you may come across better scenarios as you revise.

Chapter Four:

The 3rd Trimester - Months 7 to 9 (Weeks 28 to 40) of Pregnancy

In some ways, the third trimester is the most intense, primarily because of the extreme changes in the fetus, the mother, and the eventual onset of the actual birth. Things have become very real in an obvious way that they have not made themselves known before. The parents and everyone close to them are seeing the short ramp to the birth and beginning to anticipate the actual arrival.

However, although the finish line may appear to be insight, this is no time to let down your guard or start cheering a victory. All you have to do is look up "Premature Celebration" on YouTube. You can find all manner of examples of the tables turning when athletes give up their effort mentally before they actually achieve their end. While pregnancy isn't about winning, it is definitely about finishing the marathon, and finishing well counts whether you lead the pack or crawl in with your knees scraped as your best effort.

Your newly established fatherly habits are going to continue to carry the ball. They save mom some trouble and are something you will want to maintain. While you can look forward to a balance beginning to return sometime after the baby is born, don't count on going back to your pre-pregnancy lifestyle even then. You have taken the red pill.[1] By engaging in accepting this partnership in parenthood with your partner. There is nothing particularly scary about taking the pill, but there is no un-taking it now.

Just as before, your knowledge will prove to be influential in fielding the third trimester. If you are not surprised, you are way more prepared to handle your responsibilities well. Your reality is looking forward to the brand new experience of fatherhood and life as a dad. It will be even more of an adventure, more enduring, and likely more enjoyable than the pregnancy itself.

Time for a Review and Zapping Procrastination

If you have screwed up to this point and not paid attention to the suggestions and details for planning, you will be penalized by having to reread the whole book. Do not pass Go, do not collect an award for the best partner. Just as a 'for example,' planning would have been best to start at the turn of the first few pages. Have you started it yet? Let's see a show of hands.

Like anyone with a master's degree in procrastination, you probably have not been awarded with a trophy for being last in the class. In procrastination, he who achieves most procrastinates least. Achieving high scores in procrastination is one time where you do want to fail. You may have had one friend in high school who didn't leave every paper until the night before it was due, but my guess is that with class in session, just about every reader is going to tie at

---

[1] For those who are unfamiliar, this is a reference to the movie "The Matrix." Two pills are offered to the main character (played by Keanu Reeves), allowing him to remain in blissful ignorance or face a life-changing truth. By taking the red pill, you have done the latter.

this finish line and admit they are still putting off things they should have accomplished months ago.

Because I am aware of the propensity to procrastinate, a quick summary of what you have already learned is in order so that you start taking things a little more seriously. This review should revive your memory of what we have already covered in previous trimesters, but the review will not be repetition. Some are reviewed, but this section adds specific differences for the third trimester for each point to build on your previous goals. No playing hopscotch and jumping to the next section; these are the core values to becoming a third-trimester super dad.

Continue to Be a Partner to Your Partner

You guys have probably learned a lot about each other and learned a lot about being better partners. This part of your experience should continue to grow. Take what you have learned and expand on your skills of:

* Communications
* Recognizing her physical burden
* Staying on protection alert
* Sex and romance
* Achieving a different kind of easy

Communications. Talking about the future and continuing to nurture plans can put her mind at ease. It will make her feel that she is not alone in the practical concerns of being a new parent. Showing interest in how she feels and using your evolved communication skills will end up working out for you in the long haul. Continue to respect her motherly instincts, and don't be afraid to ask her for guidance as to what else you can do. You've got plenty of fun things to chat about. Why not start with circumcision? You'll have more of an investment in that than the color of the walls in the baby room. (See Chapter 1)

Recognize her physical burden. Nothing is getting much easier for her at this point. She is pretty much strapped to a medicine ball, and it will tax her physical skills and endurance. Eating may look like the only thing she is good at doing at times, but eating takes energy and persistence, especially when the kid you are giving a free ride to is doing their best to squish every organ you have into the size of a walnut. She might want to eat that whole pizza. She may need to eat that entire pizza. But her stomach won't accept it. Help her help herself by rising to that challenge not to feel compelled. Always be alert to ways you can genuinely help. She might get stuck on the couch and will want to get up instead of having you bring her something. Help pull her up. (See Chapters 1 and 2)

Staying on protection alert. All encounters with obvious threats to the mom and fetus should be avoided. Even if the danger of the most severe issues is lower, they have not disappeared. If you have done your job admirably, she will be feeling a little spoiled and maybe even feel entitled to certain indulgences. Still, no chewing on lead-coated pencils, engaging in toxic fine art recreation or testing out questionable herbal teas that might provide laxative effect to relieve the resident-imposed squashing of her digestive tract. As warned in a later segment of this chapter in more detail, do not let her resort to chemical removal of unusual hair growth. That is worth mentioning twice. When in doubt, consult a doctor. (See Chapter 2)

Sex and Romance. If there are no complications, sex is still a viable option and one you will want to be honest with your partner about exploring. This is no time to wrangle her into selfish advances. She may be tickled to know that her appearance has not changed the way you feel about her in any negative way. But if she is resistant, kind words and kind gestures may go as far as a lusty romp. (See Chapter 1)

Achieving a different kind of easy. You've both endured six months of the pregnancy, becoming closer through the challenges and planning for the future. In a way, the third trimester is a little like after you've done six months at a new job. It isn't new anymore. You probably both see the humor in some of the things you've learned that is now old hat. You've made it this far together, and the hindsight of rifts you might have had in more ridiculous moments are things you can laugh about. You've gone to war and come home safely. That is how bonds grow.

Review All Plans

If you have begun to plan, you haven't finished, and if you have missed planning opportunities, time to catch up. Review all your plans and amend them to incorporate what you have learned.

   * Budgeting
   * Have the birthing plan at the ready
   * Have the hospital bag at the ready

Budgeting. This is the one thing you were warned not to neglect. If you really have not looked at it and made a plan, it is imperative that the two of you sit down and go about completing the task. It is probably one of the most unpleasant things you will have to do, and it will be even more unpleasant and confusing now that you have waited this long. Do it and keep yourself from digging a financial hole, or worse. You need to cover time off, mom's needs, baby's needs, and medical costs. If you've got a plan in place, you are a champion and just need to review it and consider revisions. If not, sit down and budget now. (See Chapters 1 and 3)

Have the birthing plan at the ready. There should be a written plan that is really a ledger of doctor names, numbers, and essential information that needs to be prepared on the day of the birth so that it can be accessed easily. This can contain all the weird little details you and your partner want, like the kind of music that should be played (trust me, you won't notice who is serenading the birth). Who else is attending the actual birth can be important. The birthing room itself is not a stadium. If your mom or your partner's mom wants to be there and they are not the type you want in a war room, politely decline. This, really, optimally, is an intimate gathering of essential individuals. Your partner has to be there. If your partner wants you there, you should be. We had a nurse who was a friend of the family in attendance, and that was a great relief because she could explain all the stuff I didn't understand.

Catch the baby, or not? That's one you want to think about, dad. I absolutely refused. If anybody was dropping anything, it wasn't going to be me, regardless of my fielding percentage in baseball. I'd never heard the end of it. On a scale of 1-10, how much do you want to avoid an episiotomy? On a scale of 1-10, where do you weigh in on epidural? Some of these things will fade from your control because that's why doctors are in the room. But you want to get your preferences down. If you started the plan months ago, bravo, my brave knight! Now update it with everything you thought of afterwards.

The unwritten plan should also be ready. That is mostly a daddy-do where you take a hospital tour, know the route and alternates, and plan for unforeseen circumstances. One of your most important jobs is to keep gas in the car all the time. I used to have a habit of flirting with how close the needle could get to the letter 'E' on the gas gauge without running out. During the period of the final trimesters, I was keeping my car full, and when I got home, I'd check my partner's car just in case. (See Chapter 1)

Have the hospital bag at the ready. On the day of the awaited event, you don't want to be fishing for your toothbrush or anything else that you'll need during your hospital stay. If you have not put the bag together, do it now and tick it off the list. You cannot count on precisely nine months or 40 weeks being right to the day. This bag is at the ready by week 30, or you are neglecting your responsibilities. (See Chapter 1)

Don't Neglect Yourself.

You may not be the primary player, but if one of the members of the team goes down, it isn't going to be you. You need to be there to help hold her up and keep her pushing toward your next adventure of parenthood. The only way you will do that is by being of sound mind and body. To that end, you need to:

* Stay fit, alert, and maintain friendships
* Watch the weight gain
* Breathe and meditate

Stay fit, alert, and maintain friendships. The most significant change you would want to make from the original outline of taking time for yourself is taking time for both of you. She may feel less motivated to maintain any exercise regimen simply because it is harder and more uncomfortable to move. Choose light exercises like walking or ask to participate in things you notice she might not be doing anymore. Saying something like: "Can you teach me some yoga that you've been practicing?" puts her in the position of being the expert, and she may like that. Encouragement is the key. The last thing you want is for her to lack the stamina she needs for childbirth because you dropped the ball in motivating her. You also don't want to get a call from the hospital while you are out at a pub with friends that the baby came early. 'Congratulations,' you missed the entire experience you've been waiting nine months for. It won't be worth it. (See Chapter 1 and 2)

Watch the weight gain. There is a suggested range of weight that women should stay within during pregnancy. There is also a warning for men. While women gain weight during pregnancy, men usually do, too. The odd trade-off is that a bunch of the weight she is gaining is somebody else's, and yours is all you. According to various sources, men gain an average of 15 pounds from being exposed to new snack opportunities, eating out more, and eating for two, even when there is only one. Along with staying fit, stay aware of extra calories you are allowing yourself that you shouldn't, and maybe make it up in some other way. You can pack smaller lunches for work and knock off fewer Friday beers. (See Chapter 2)

Breathe and meditate. This is another potential group activity that will accomplish a different goal in the final trimester. If you have successfully incorporated breathing exercises and meditation into your routine, helping your partner practice can provide another weapon against the trials, persistence, and rigors of childbirth. It is a stressful time and getting mom to be able to create self-imposed calm may quell what can be self-defeating anxiety. There's no way to guarantee stress-reducing regimens will have the baby drop out with greater ease, but as long as the practice is not extreme, it may help you contribute in a meaningful way to the experience in the birthing room. (See Chapter 2)

Further Your Education

Of course, you haven't learned everything yet. That will come your second time around when you can look at the first one and say: "He told me in the book, and I just didn't pay attention." Next, we are taking a brief look at some topics and specific concerns that may not yet be in the scope of your radar.

* Utilize your experience resources
* Pertussis vaccine
* Kick-starting labor

Utilize your experience resources. I didn't exactly say this in the introduction, but having no experience with a baby will mean you have none. Changing a real baby is nothing like changing a dummy. Holding an actual child will test those skills and give you valuable experience you can build on. If you have friends and relatives with kids and infants, being around them can help your education. The difference between before — when you wondered why people had to ruin a perfectly good BBQ with a bunch of brats — and now, is that you will soon be the one ruining the BBQ. That's not the entirety of it. Now you have a vested interest in paying attention to how others parent so you can learn from them. Up to this point, other people's kids were like so many flies landing on the burgers or wasps hovering around the grill. Now they are your little teachers. Watch what makes them not cry. Select from the menu of things you will and won't do with your own kid. Hold babies. Friends and family will be amused and glad to offer advice. Don't drop the baby.

Pertussis vaccine. In some countries, the Pertussis vaccine is recommended for all pregnant women sometime between the 16th and 32nd weeks of pregnancy. Getting vaccinated during this period allows for the antibodies to be passed from the mother to the fetus with reliable transmission time. These vaccines provide protection against whooping cough, polio, tetanus, and diphtheria (there are some variants to the Boostrix IPV vaccine, so it is best to ask your doctor specifically which variant he will be using). Whooping cough is the primary reason for the vaccine. Babies who get whooping cough often require hospitalization, and the vaccine effectively prevents whooping cough in 91% of cases studied since 2012. Studies have shown little to no side effects besides very minor redness, swelling or tenderness for mom as might happen with any injection. The vaccine is optional, and with the swirl of misinformation about vaccination due to COVID social media doctors and misinformed anti-vaxers, there is probably more resistance to vaccinations now than ever. This is despite the overwhelming good vaccines have done for the health and welfare of humanity. Unless either the mother or the father has had some type of severe allergic reaction to a vaccine, there is virtually no reason to have any concerns about taking it. Much better to do this than to risk a potentially fatal hospitalization stay for pneumonia.

Kick-starting labor. There is a lot of information on Google about things that will help start labor. Some are simple and seem not to be dangerous, and others are reckless and ridiculous. The things to try if you need to are harmless ones which include having sex, exercising, nipple stimulation, acupressure, and eating certain foods (pineapple, dates, eggplant, spicy food, etc.). If what you are eating is not weird and in amounts that can be toxic to mom or fetus, it may at least satisfy you that you are trying to get the ball rolling. It would be hard to say that you are doing anything by the time it gets to this point. Whatever seems successful may just be a coincidence as you won't be working at starting the engine before the due date anyway. In our first run, my wife and I were sitting on the couch watching something like "America's Funniest Home Videos," and someone got their tongue stuck on an ice-cube tray. We both started laughing, and then she blurted, "get me a towel!!" There was nothing in me asking why by this point. I ran to the closet and brought back assorted colors. Then we grabbed the hospital bags, hopped in the car, and we were off to the hospital. I sort of like that it happened with a laugh.

The idea of inducing labor is something else entirely. When you get to around week 42, and the contractions still have not begun to convert to labor, the doctor will let you know it is time to induce. It is probably best that you leave decisions of this magnitude up to the experts in the long run. However, it is also good to keep in mind that there is a bit of a downside to inducing labor. Recovery tends to be slower. It is impossible to say if that is directly related to the induction or just because the pregnancy is on overtime. The other thing is that contractions can be more intense, as can be the pain of labor. This may be a reason to add a clause to your birthing plan along the line of "If induced, then epidural."

Immersing Yourself in Understanding Trimester #3

While many things may seem to have become routine over time, it is evident that other things keep changing virtually by the day. The one thing that may not be subject to change is you; the hope is you have successfully formed yourself into a rock of consistency, improved as a human, and you are tipping the scales measuring the applause for your performance. You still need to keep your radar on what's going on.

* What is happening with the baby?
* What's happening with your partner?
* How can you best be of help?

What is going on with the baby? Until this trimester, the baby has been doing more to grow in length than in girth. The baby will bulk up almost 50% over the trimester, and that comes in the way of organ development and shaping into what you recognize as a newborn. The eyes will open somewhere around week 28, and the fine hairs that have been protecting the skin for the past months will begin to shed. Right about week 35, the baby will shift its squished position so that its head will point down in order to exit head-first. It doesn't always happen, and that is considered a 'breach baby,' affecting about 5% of births. It can lead to complications, but it is really not a major concern in a situation with well-trained staff (doctors tend to be well-trained).

One of the most important things that will be going on throughout the trimester is the development of the lungs. One of the reasons premature babies have a rough time is that breathing is an issue because the lungs do not have the chance to form fully.

Development goes on throughout the trimester; that is why it is best to go full-term. Even if mom is a little tired of being a free ride, she should not be doing anything to promote early labor unless at the suggestion of her physician.

The baby sleeps about 90% of the time and can REM sleep and dream. While sleeping most of the time, that does not mean there will be a lot of inactivity. Just like watching your dog chasing imaginary rabbits through the underbrush, the baby may exhibit activity even while sleeping. The baby will be practicing many things that will come in handy when finally escaping their holiday chamber. They may be smiling, frowning, and crying, and essentially taking baby steps in their development.

What is happening with your partner? Until this point, there hasn't been a tremendous amount of stuff you've needed to know about your partner that you can participate in beyond lending a helping hand and exhibiting patience. Things change here as much more becomes obvious, and your partner's personality starts to play into her role as bun bearer. She may be frustrated with all the things which make her experience technical difficulties as if the little darling on the inside is pulling marionette strings on the outside.

It is tough to say just how the 'little lady' is feeling at this point about going from however little she was to however big she has gotten. The average weight gain during pregnancy is about 30 pounds, including the baby (and other things that rapidly exit during the birth). This weight gain can present in various ways, such as enlarged breasts, fat reserves, and blood and fluid volumes. The frame of the mother before the pregnancy will matter when it comes to total distortion, as will any special diets. My mother was a small woman who miraculously gained only 15 pounds during pregnancy, and I was almost 10 of those. When the birth was over, besides reminding me forever that I almost killed her for the next 45 years, she was looking about the same as before she got pregnant the day after I was born. That is not normal, and the excuse was that she was on a special, precautionary diet which somehow had absolutely no effect on my growth but was critical for survival.

You don't want to try and have your partner mimic that performance because it is unlikely. However, you do want to pay attention to the expected range for gain. Your doctor will likely tell you what that range should be and will issue a warning if mom goes off the rails. In general, petite women should gain much more, both by percentage and in total, than women who are already a bit on the plump side.

These changes may be distressing to moms who are not used to seeing themselves with extra weight. My spouse was tiny all her life. Born at 2.7 kilos (just under 6 pounds) at full term, she held to just 43 kilos (95 pounds) without change over the ages of 18 to 31. As her athletic body started to morph because of the pregnancy, she knew she needed just to accept it. A week before birth, she weighed in at a 'monstrous' (for her) 61 kilos (about 135 pounds). In other words, she came up to the top end of the average for her height for women who were not pregnant. There was 50% more of her to love. Somehow her metabolism managed to knock almost all of what survived the birth back off her frame in record time. Her experience was nearly the polar opposite of my mother, although the baby size was similar. In all, the safe thing to say is that the experience will be different for every woman.

What the fantastic final third of incubation does manage to do is distress the pregnant partner in one way or another — and likely several ways at the same time. Pre-pregnancy framing and metabolism play a part in where everything gets squished too. Especially at the end of the trimester, it is safe to say that any woman's framework will be like a balloon inflated to just that point where no more air can go in. Then the baby is going to try as it might to just get those few more tiny puffs in, or else it isn't really testing the quality of its ride. Your job is primarily to stay aware that mom will be uncomfortable.

Wacky stuff goes on, and some of it is really interesting. Other parts leading up to the ultimate event may just seem a little gross depending on your level of tolerance. Some can even be a little frightening. You can think it, but don't say it. Try not to make faces either. You want to keep your meter dead center between "Oh, it's nothing" and "I'm calling 911" at all times. Accept that things will present and you haven't seen them before. It's sort of like having the doorbell ring and knowing when you open it up, you are either going to see an alien or not. Best to try and look at it all with wonder rather than trepidation and assume all aliens come in peace.

Several things present in ways that will be pretty apparent. While her normal head of hair may seem even more lush and beautiful, she may start to grow hair in places that she might not particularly care for — like her face, nipples, and back. This is most likely an annoyance that will reverse after the birth. Do not let her use chemical treatments of any sort to defeat this strike to her vanity. If it absolutely drives her bonkers and there is a need to attend to her vanity, offer to help her out, but always be kind and supportive if you do. Depending on your relationship, she might prefer that a friend's hand be put to the task of depilation.

Some cute can happen in the manifestation of body-in-change besides just the omnipresent belly bubble. Her belly button may pop if she does not already sport an outtie. Her areola may darken and change shape and size, which is thought to be so that baby will have an easier time locating and latching on. Breasts can also vary in various ways, usually to enlarge and become more firm. Regretfully they may be sore sometimes, which may have started even before the diagnosis of pregnancy way back in week 1 or 2. By the third trimester, the aches and pains of becoming engorged may make the largeness of her breasts seem even more enticing than usual. Careful there, bucko! You may like what you see, but it may not be the best time to display your affection. Remain conscious that they may be particularly tender. On the other hand, you only really have to avoid sex if 1) she is not interested, 2) everything is not progressing normally. If her water breaks or there is another discharge, use good sense and hold off for a more reasonable time.

During this trimester it may seem that every part of her has been injected with a little gremlin and wants to have the opportunity to complain. For example, even the most athletic of the female species is likely to experience some form of shortness of breath. This may be more noticeable to those who have particularly good habits of breathing from the diaphragm. As there is no longer much space for the diaphragm to move downward, breathing may be more shallow. Of course, this is complicated by the fact that she is breathing for two. Reminders to maintain good posture over slouching can actually relieve some of these symptoms while regretfully calling for additional resources that she may feel she has run out of.

The squish-squashing and extra weight assembled in such a short term may mean a change in an exercise regimen. Very low impact aerobic efforts like walking and exercise classes, especially for pregnant women, may be just the thing. Don't wait for her to figure out what she needs, and be on the lookout for opportunities such as public pool memberships where you can accompany her to work out with recommended regimens together. Don't, don't, don't go at it like a viper because she might think you are insulting her new curves and are overly concerned with the way she looks. Always keep the context of partnership and baby welfare. If going the public pool route, check reviews to ensure the facility has an impeccable reputation for cleanliness and safety. Besides the obvious exercises for flexibility and fitness, she should probably be doing kegel (pelvic floor) workouts several times a day. You can help with reminders. These can help during birth and may yield other benefits in recovery and return to a somewhat enhanced sex life when all is done.

She may complain of vague numbness or pain in the lower back, butt, and shooting pains that radiate down her leg. This is her sciatic nerve complaining about the pressure on it because it too is being squeezed. Warm compresses, simple massage devices (or her partner's gentle hand), exercise, or even just changing positions can all contribute to relief. In moments where it becomes intense, some pain killers might be considered as a last resort. Be sure to check with the doctor before ingesting anything, especially if it is a miracle cure found on some suspicious website or in a well-meaning YouTube video.

Mom may experience premature contractions, known as Braxton Hicks contractions. It is probably best to just think of these as practice for the real thing. They can come on in various ways but will most likely be something like a cramp, a solid muscle contraction that mom is not doing intentionally. Of course, it is possible that labor can start prematurely, and it is best to be able to know the difference. Braxton Hicks contractions are irregular, and if there are clusters, they tend to get weaker. Often they can be relaxed just by changing position (standing up, walking, etc.). Real contractions will not just be clusters that dissipate. They will keep coming in waves and will tend to get stronger. While that is still a bit vague, contractions for actual labor will come every 5 minutes, lasting one minute, for at least one hour. This may be accompanied by a discharge (e.g., water breaking). In other words, you need to take contractions seriously when they seem insistent, or like the last guest at a party that gets on the phone and calls some people to come over to liven things up a bit when the party sputters out.

The baby is active and kicking. There will be significant downtime, but there will be moments where the baby will seem to be trying to break out of the shell-like it is in an egg with limbs flying nearly like a kickboxer. How easy these are actually to observe on a bare belly will come down to fat reserves that have been stored, but they will be apparent to the touch. The doctor may suggest monitoring baby movements just to track the frequency to ensure everything continues to progress nicely.

Mother's trips to the doctor will increase to about every two weeks and may be as frequent as once a week as the trimester comes to a close. Always attend when you can, and when you can't, be sure someone goes with her. Can she go by herself? Sure. She is probably doing a lot of things by herself. Living humans will be like that, and especially if she is feeling perky, there's no reason she can't be alone. But give me a good reason why.

One thing she may be spending some particular amount of time within a variety of different ways is deliberate forms of nesting. This can be in the form of cleaning and preparing, fussing with the arrangement of baby things, watching cooking shows, reading about taking care of newborns, watching programming that seems peculiar to her normal regimen, etc. This more likely has to do with embracing the mindset of being a mom and having had nine months to appreciate that she is already responsible for the life of an entirely new human. Soon it will be kicking and screaming and laughing and being adorable in what seems more like real-time. Common sense says: "You've got to be ready; it's showtime."

The Pet Aside

If you have pets, they likely will have become aware of the fact that something is going on. Either cats or dogs will probably sense changes that humans just do not have the ability to. They won't want to be left out of the family event, and really they shouldn't be. You want to do as little to surprise them with a new

---

alien and change their lifestyle as little as possible. The final word here is to take care of the pet, acclimating it to the situation and being sure that it will embrace the intruder who will be nabbing significant companionship time.

Practice taking the dog for a walk with an empty stroller if possible, so they are prepared for the real thing. If you can't get the dog to be your partner in walks with the carriage, now is the time to find out. It is better to watch them knock the thing over when it is unoccupied than when the buggy contains a precious cargo, and you'll have to contend with a baby rolling out onto the concrete. It may give you an idea of whether you can take care of two walks at one time or if you are forced to take two walks. An alternative is to hire a dog walker.

After the actual birth, it may be advisable to bring home something with the baby's scent from the hospital to create that familiarity before introducing the baby to the house. Surprise is not always the best means of introduction. No matter how acutely aware the pet may be or how intelligent, everything you can do to ease the transition is just another measure of smart parenting.

Cats will probably have made themselves more critically aware of being attracted to the cozy warmth mom is exuding. Just a reminder to keep mom clear of kitty litter as toxoplasmosis is never a good thing during pregnancy.

More care may be needed with exotic pets than typical domestics. It is best to keep any type of rodent away from baby (and mom) as they may carry a virus called lymphocytic choriomeningitis which can cause serious complications. Lizards, snakes, turtles, and other amphibians may carry salmonella and listeria monocytogenes. While you may have a deep emotional attachment to pets, you do not want to risk introducing the baby to a bacterium and have to rationalize the relative importance. In some instances, it may be best to face the facts and get that exotic critter out of the house entirely.

How can you help? You got this far, and you know it isn't over. Getting this far taught you a lot of things, and you are ready to push through. You have got to be the one who picks up the pieces that fall on the ground because a few months enter here that she won't see her own toes when standing in the shower. You have to review what you learned, review the plans, check, double-check, and step in to be the cavalry on call.

When you learn martial arts, the idea is not violence but a calm, natural reaction. When you go to break a board, you don't aim to do it by hitting the board because that's how you break your own bones. You want to strike an inch or more beyond the immediate target, so everything you have goes right through. You are not looking at the water breaking, the labor pains, the trip to the hospital, or even the baby's first gasping breath as the end. You have to stay on task past there and be a pillar of your new family. You'll remember your effort, and you'll do better next time if you have the chance. Your partner will have all the focus will get all the attention and credit, but she will also know that you did it together. Just like "behind every great man, there is a great woman," this is the opposite side of the coin.

Punch through that barrier.

Parenting and Partnering Power

You really have to corral the last-minute obligations going into the final stretch. You want nothing to be up in the air by the end of this trimester as you are getting down to game time. The home needs to be ready for the new arrival, and all your plans should be in place. If you have been working on them even a few minutes a week and doing monthly reviews, everything should be in pretty good order. Don't let that fool you. Keep up with what you know you have to do.

This trimester can be a time of bonding like you, and your partner will not have it again for a long time. You'll see the humor in things that were worrisome in the first two trimesters, the goal will feel like it is insight, and it will probably be easier to inject some well-intended humor into things that you may have been too nervous about joking about before. Keep to your regimens, and don't lie to your notebook. It knows. Stay rested, fit, and ready, and give yourself some credit for becoming a better partner.

Chapter Five:

The Fourth Trimester

While technically not part of pregnancy, the period following the birth is a time of significant adjustment. It is hard to put a period at the end of pregnancy and say it is all over as far as the dad's participation is concerned. In fact, it's not hard. It's wrong.

A book for dads about pregnancy would be remiss not to cover what happens in the few months following birth. It may not be fitting to extend too far into the future as that is the subject of a different book. Certainly, the period where your baby was not breathing the same air as you has passed, and the wriggling squirming bundle is out in the physical world. It is a new leg of the journey, but the following steps forward are like the close of a movie after the climax, which ends with a clever denouement, and you end up satisfied and looking forward to the sequel.

In case it hasn't sunk in, you are officially a dad now. The physical burden that mainly was the responsibility of your partner has arrived, now is the time you can do some actual sharing of the physical child. Your family now has three members, for better or worse, and you are headed on a new leg of the journey.

What Happened in the Delivery Room

Because you paid attention to all the planning and details laid out in this book, your hospital experience during the birth went swimmingly. The water broke, you hopped in the car, and you made it to the Emergency Room doors without running a single red light even though you had to track around a water-main burst. Your partner was admitted, and you parked the car in under a minute and were back by her side in three. The birthing plan was followed to a "T", and — boom — out came baby without any effort. If you are paying attention to the sarcasm, that is likely not what happened.

Labor may have lasted far longer than you expected. The average is about 8 hours. You only think it is a lot quicker because of what you see on TV or in movies. Do you know why labor goes quickly when produced as part of a film? That's called drama and allowed storytime. Movies can't take eight hours to show a woman going through all the pains of labor, and it would blow their budget and the box office if they did. The people who are really invested in the birthing room are the parents living the real drama and the good people seeing them successfully through the experience.

Our first-time labor was a total of 16 hours. Things on the birthing plan did not pan out exactly, and probably neither will yours. Your regular doctor may have had three patients go into labor simultaneously, so while they may have been in contact with whoever filled in for them, they may not have made the actual delivery, especially if they work in more than one hospital. Your partner may have kept her head through the stress and pain, or she may have turned into someone you had never met before whose hand you were trying to hold while she slapped it away with a poly-syllabic swear. You may both have become delirious from sleep deprivation, and the baby was just beginning to show the incredible ability to misunderstand the word "cooperation."

Hopefully, you were able to stand by your end of the bargain, fight through dizzy spells and unexpected moments. Hopefully, the birthing plan eased you and your partner's navigation through the hours of delivery. Even if the plan said you'd cut the cord and you opted out while slightly overwhelmed, that doesn't make the plan a failure — and neither are you. The plan made sure you thought things through and knew the way it was supposed to go. Like a wedding, something always pops up to defeat what should have been perfect planning. It could be rain, the flower truck crashing, or the best man's phone battery dying, but in the end, the show must go on. At the very least, you've got this maiden voyage off your list of to-dos, and you will become world-wise from the event. Should you have the opportunity to experience it again, you will be better prepared, but things will still head off in unexpected directions in encore presentations.

Inevitably, somewhat frightening, things may have happened. More likely than not, these would only be frightening because you were not in on the details. My first child put me through some bit of unexpected trauma by arriving in a bluish tint and not taking what I thought would be the quick gulp of isopropyl-scented hospital air. Minutes before the birth, the doctor told me that there were some complications with an entangled cord and that really it wasn't much to worry about. Well, I took the advice and didn't worry, but that didn't exactly tell me what to expect. An entangled umbilical cord occurs in nearly a quarter of all pregnancies, making it fairly common. Just how it is entangled and where can make the potential result more complicated. If the cord is wrapped loosely somewhere, there may be almost no presentation or issues. If it is tightly wrapped somewhere, the entanglement may choke off the flow of the baby's nourishment through the cord as well as affect the baby's circulation to the brain. Of course, doctors who have seen this hundreds or thousands of times are not about to panic.

I saw my blue baby put on a cart after the cord was cut, limp, and silent, and I knew better beforehand not to participate in 'catching the baby' or 'cutting the cord.' Someone else's kid, no problem, but not my own. I watched as a nurse kept looking up at the wall clock.

The nurse walked round and round the baby cleaning things up and rubbing her feet, and all I could think was, "It's dead." It wasn't nearly the expected outcome, and I couldn't even look at my partner. No one said another thing to me as they were all set to tasks of tending mom, baby, supplies, and machinery as if infant mortality was no concern at all. There is where my education about childbirth failed. What seemed to me to be an interminable time between the baby's arrival and the first breath was no more than three minutes in reality. Time has a different meaning in stressful situations, especially for those who are stressed. The cord had indeed been choking her, but some quick moves by the physician in charge eased the baby's arrival and sped her to the cart. While I stood a few feet away, ready to barge in and slap the baby myself as I'd seen done so often on TV, that the first yelp sung out spontaneously, and baby blue pinked up in short order. Moments later, we were informed it was a girl (Yes, we actually chose not to know if it were a boy or a girl), and I was invited to visit the cart when I would no longer be in the way of people doing their jobs. Not to blame the doctor doing the delivery, but if she had just said, "the baby may be a little off-color and may not breathe right away," I'd have avoided that brief meltdown. But it isn't every doctor's job to present a class. I should have read that. Aside from the nurse looking up at the clock, no one was doing anything that showed concern. There were no machines being wheeled in, no respirator, no whispering huddles. I'd come to the game under-prepared.

As it turns out, there is about a 10-minute window before the baby will potentially experience more severe issues and much longer before the issue of mortality arises. Her initial APGAR was four, which I actually did know was in the range of moderately abnormal, and my personal education had gotten me that far. I knew that four was not the kind of number you wanted to hear, and I didn't know which things she was earning points for. Had I not been so panicked, I would have realized that she was getting zero points for appearance, zero for activity, and zero for respiration, but that also meant her little heart must have been beating. She was earning points for something I couldn't see from where I was standing (see the APGAR Scores sidebar). The happy part of the story is that once she took that first breath, her score jumped to eight, and the immediate danger fluttered away on the same wings on which it came. A lesson to learn here is that probably everyone in the room knows more about what is going on than you do. It's no sin to ask a question. Keep them to a minimum, and don't be a pest. Never tell your doctors what to do unless they ask your opinion.

APGAR Scores

APGAR stands for Appearance, Pulse, Grimace, Activity, and Respiration. The scores are a means of quickly evaluating a baby's relative health. The evaluations can be done several times, from immediately after birth through an extended period if there seems to be some concern. The rating is based on five categories where the baby can score from 0 to 2 for each category, with the highest score being a ten. The categories and points include:

* Appearance (0 — The baby is blue, 1 — the baby has blue hands or feet, 2 — the baby is pink)
* Pulse (0 — Below 60 beats per minute, 1 — 60 to 100 beats per minute, 2 — greater than 100 beats per minute)
* Grimace (0 — No response to stimulation, 1 — slight reaction to stimulation 2 — a clear reaction to stimulation)
* Respiration (0 — Not breathing, 1 — weak cry, 2 — strong cry)
* Muscle tone (0 — Limp, 1 — reserved motion, 2 — active motion)

The most confusing of these is 'Grimace.' All it means is that the baby reactsto a reflexive stimulus like a gentle pinch or another discomfort. This is hardly high science and does not require medical tools.

The test is given routinely immediately after the birth and then again five minutes after. If the five-minute test still shows an APGAR of less than seven, the score may continue to be monitored for an extended time.

We had three surprises during the birth, a late epidural (my partner wanted to avoid pain relief entirely because of potential risks), an episiotomy (once almost considered standard procedure and now used far less often, it was not on the birthing plan), and the wayward cord. My wife took the epidural as a last-minute call when she was offered the final opportunity (some doctors will do epidurals right up to the moment of crowning). The good part about waiting was there was less chance of affecting the baby because the time between the epidural being introduced and the actual birth was fairly short. The risk to mother and child is relatively low, but complications can arise.

You may have had a moment or two when you faltered as I did, but imagine how much worse that could have been if you had not been as well prepared. If you went a little woozy at the sight of some things that went on, hopefully, you hid it from your partner as her lady parts went through calisthenics that you never dreamed were possible. Your birthing plan should have included just how close you get to the action. If you know you get wobbly knees at the sight of blood, it might be best to stand north of the center of activity as you try to comfort your partner, or just stand back or even out of the room if it is not the place for you.

Other Birthing Options

It is probably true to say no one plans on a cesarian. That will probably be your doctor's call in response to some complication that is not easily resolved in another way. Obviously, this is a surgical procedure and will require a more hands-on deck. The prep and procedure will probably not take more than 30 minutes, but it complicates recovery time.

Mom will have to be placed on fluids and pain killers, which would not usually be necessary after natural childbirth. While it may not be the preferred option, just be glad it is available and accept that it was the best advice given to you. Be aware that c-section rates vary from hospital to hospital and doctor to doctor. You may want to enquire long in advance about the record of your ob-gyn and hospital.

Induced labor will be much like natural birth except with the preamble. There is no real surprise of the water breaking and unexpected contractions unless, by coincidence, normal labor starts on the induction day. It should end up being more like attending a doctor's appointment without any mad dash to the ER. This is usually an option used when the due date is overdue. Several ways of speeding things along include an Oxytocin drip, cervical ripening with prostaglandin (which relaxes the cervix through a vaginal application), and stripping membranes. One or more methods might be used depending on the difficulty of starting the engine or the reason for the induction. For the most part, induction will be the same as natural childbirth except that it is generally accepted to be faster and more intense (I.e., painful).

In all, your job as a partner remains about the same while the medical professionals go about their work. Good for you if you performed your role well. If there were chinks in the armor, learn from your mistakes.

Immersing Yourself in Understanding a Successful Birth

   * What is happening with the baby?
   * What's happening with your partner?
   * How can you best be of help?

What is happening with the baby? Baby just got plopped out of its comfortable, warm nest into the bright lights and big city of a hospital room. It is a lot to get used to when compared to the muffled, dull plodding of the womb. No wonder most of them start crying almost immediately. The baby is tended to with any special care concerns, but mostly the focus will be on acclimating the child to mom and the new real world. The baby will be weighed and measured, given antibiotic eye drops, and a shot of vitamin K. The latter helps normalize blood clotting. They will take the baby's footprints for records and additional ID.

Before even leaving the birthing room, mom, dad, and baby will all get ID bracelets that they need to have at all times to be sure the parents are reunited with the correct children. The goal is to make the nightmare of a potential mixup something that is nearly impossible. There were tragic records in the past of babies being swapped at birth, but gladly the practice has evolved. In extreme cases, DNA could be used to identify the proper parents of a child.

Post-birth tests include hearing tests, blood tests, and observation for congenital heart defects. If required, the baby may be tested for HIV and hepatitis. If it is a boy and the option for circumcision is selected, it may be performed within the first two days. A practice becoming more common is having parents return after a week or two for the procedure.

Once you are out of the hospital, the baby no longer has the automated support system and protection of the mother's body. The hospital staff will not trail you home, and the baby is totally dependent on its parents for survival. Intending to that level of care, neither parent is likely to get a lot of sleep, and that will remain the case for some time until things settle into a routine.

What's happening with your partner? Your partner just went through a sudden colossal change in her physique. She might be the type just to shrug it off, or she may find the shift somewhat disorienting. She may be superhuman if she isn't at least a little light-headed, extremely relieved, or even giddy immediately after the birth.

Mom and baby will remain in recovery for two to four days, depending on whether it was natural childbirth or not. This may vary due to hospital policies. Regardless, mom's body will have to begin a process of repair. She needs to eat healthily, stay hydrated, and care for her state until her strength returns.

Rely on her to choose whether or not to accept visitors. People may have stayed in the waiting room hoping to hear the good news, but that does not mean they should automatically be admitted after birth to be the first to see the baby. Your partner will likely be exhausted, not feeling that she looks her best (despite and because of the sudden loss of 15 pounds), or may just need some downtime to get it in her head that the process is complete. She will probably be happy to have fewer doctors poking and prodding as if she were a science experiment and learning how to be a new mom is the premiere item on her list.

Breastfeeding is new to her, and the first attempts may be as soon as an hour after birth. There can be issues here as likely as not with the baby learning mom's anatomy and mom having zero experience. Hospitals will likely have a specialist on staff to consult for breastfeeding issues. It is important for mother and child to have that time to bond.

There are likely to be mood swings brought on by exhaustion, hormones, and simple emotional reactions to reality. Joy, disbelief, even missing having her baby inside her can come on her in a moment. The fluctuations may wear off in just a few weeks or may linger. In extreme cases, it may evolve into post-partum depression. Suspicion of the latter should be evaluated. In all, the hope is that things gradually return to normal for her and you over the next six weeks or so. Be her careful watchman, and don't assume it is time to leave your post.

How you can help. Your role as a father has completely changed when the baby emerges from the womb. You are not a player on the sidelines just tending to your partner (and yourself), but there is a list of new tasks and skills to develop. These will be things you already know we're on the way. Still, your previous experience with all of them has more likely been in the form of a fire drill than a fire (unless you did as suggested and explored your personal resources to get experience with actual babies).

The hands-on skills that you need to acquire include the following, and almost exactly in this order:

* Holding the baby
* Getting the baby in a car seat
* Diaper changing
* Feeding the baby
* Burping the baby
* Putting the baby to bed

Holding the Baby. Your baby is nothing like sporting equipment. The package is quite delicate and more like a priceless urn than a football. Newborns don't have much stamina, muscle, or coordination, and especially during the first two months, you want to pay particular care to support the neck and head. Keep in mind that said 'particular care.' The whole package requires your attention. You don't want to approach the situation with fear, but you really need to exhibit mindful gentility.

Until your baby shows significant ability to support the weight of their own head, it is literally in your hands to do it for them. When lifting the baby, always support the neck and head with one hand and the baby's bottom with the other. It may take a little practice to transfer to the cradle hold, but even for many dads, this will come naturally. As the baby gets older (over three months and supports the weight of their own head comfortably), you can experiment with other holds that will be more comfortable for you and the child.

Holding the baby will be something you will experience before you leave the hospital, whether someone hands you the child or if you go to pick it up on your own. Always err on the side of caution the first few times you hold your newborn, and don't be shy about asking questions or advice, and listen when it is offered. No one wants to tell a new dad it looks like it is his first time to the skating rink. Comments are made to help you and secure the welfare of your child.

Getting the Baby in a Car Seat. The next thing I am sure I did was awkwardly get my child into a car seat. I'd yet to leave the hospital parking lot, and after successfully managing to not dump her out of the carrier, I then managed to successfully maneuver her into place with the seat facing the rear of the car. I would swear this was only possible because I'd already put the seat in and taken it out a dozen times in practice. Do not make the mistake of thinking you'll just figure out the seat on the day you bring the baby home. While people picture the ride from the hospital to their residence as some type of fairy tale, if it happens to be pouring rain or the hottest day of the summer, you won't want to spend a lot of time reading instructions you forgot to bring. If it is that steamy hot day, be sure to cool down the car before getting the baby down. She might like to be swaddling warm, but she won't much like roasting in an oven.

Our hospital had a policy that a specialist would come out to watch me install the seat and be sure I got it right. It may be possible to request this service if it is not offered as standard practice. There's another gem to get on the Unwritten Plan. You do not want a simple pump on the brakes to spill your special cargo just because you didn't put in the time to get it right.

Diaper Changing. While you may have the opportunity to change your baby for the first time at the hospital, your first time may likely be at the homestead with the luxury of a dedicated changing table. If that is the case, someone smarter than you has probably stocked the area with all the practical things you will need at one point or another to address the mess. It is inevitable that you will forget something and that your first few changes should be monitored. After just a couple, you will develop all the skills you need to improvise quick-thinking solutions to what-the-heck moments. Supplies may run out, and the baby will not have the courtesy to wait to do anything while in the midst of a change. Think of supplies like toilet paper and always replace the roll when it runs out.

In those more special moments where you learn that a diaper can weigh as much as the baby (or so it seems), you will keep your cool and manage to deal with the most prominent mountains of poop while leaving the area spotless and the baby free of diaper rash. Learn what you really need and wrap your head around the moments you have to pack the travel bag yourself. That time will come.

Feeding the Baby. Of course, if mom is breastfeeding, your participation in baby nourishment will be limited as far as the role you can play. However, when and if mom plans to go back to work, you pull split shifts or merely want to do your part to let your partner sleep, you have to be capable and knowledgeable about feeding the baby. Formula or milk that has been pumped and stored in the fridge should be brought up to the proper temperature. It isn't actually necessary to heat formula, but if you consider the original source, the freshest supply of milk with being about 98.6 degrees. The word 'about' is in there to acknowledge the fact that breasts may not be precisely average temperature because not all people are. They are also often wrapped in extra garments and extend from the torso, so it is hard to say one way or another that there is a perfect temperature. It does, however, seem counter-intuitive to provide the baby with something they might find less comforting and satisfying by sticking them with a cold liquid diet.

Be careful not to overheat the milk. It is not a bad idea to use a double boiler. You can even just heat a bottle in a pot of warm water. Just run warm water off the tap and place the bottle in. No matter how you do it, always check the final temperature of the milk. Some mysterious force might be at work to thwart your best efforts. Make sure the milk is mixed well by tipping the bottle a few times end-over-end and putting a squirt on your wrist. That isn't an exact science either, so err on the safe side.

When using powdered formula and mixing your own, you want to ensure that the water source is pure and does not contain high amounts of chemicals commonly found in tap water like fluoride and chlorine. In cases where you are using well water, it is probably best to boil the water first for several minutes and allow it to cool. In most cases, tap water should be safe, but it may be advisable to take extra care depending on where you live. If using bottled water, check the ratings on purity. It won't be within everyone's budget to install a purification system, but even those will vary in effectiveness and viability.

Ensure that all formula or breast milk is stored correctly, and take care to observe limitations as to how long you leave it out. It is far from impossible that you can create unsafe conditions for milk storage, especially when you are out and about with a travel bag. Be careful about promptly emptying bottles that have been used and keep things clean if not absolutely sterile. No one likes this sentence, but: read the manufacturer's instructions for handling all bottle-feeding equipment!

Burping the Baby. One thing that dads can probably relate to is a baby's need to burp. If the gas stays down when you eat too fast or knock back a carbonated beverage, it just means you'll be uncomfortable. Well, that goes for baby too. Air that slips by the suckling is going to be uncomfortable, and until it bursts free from entrapment, it is cause for discomfort at nap time and crying jags.

What you are trying to do in burping is create an environment where tiny bubbles in the tiny belly merge so they can escape in one whopping yodel. The favored methods are tapping the baby's back just below the shoulder blades or rubbing. The result is the same thing: introducing gentle vibrations encourages the bubbles to merge. Please note the word 'gentle' as key to success and avoiding anything more abrupt that might be considered shaking the baby.

The easiest way for most new dads to do this is to throw a burp nap (also more notoriously known as a vomit rag) over your shoulder and then cradle the baby's bottom in the right arm to face toward your chest and toward the rag. Spend some time tapping and rubbing the baby's back. The bubbles will collect and escape.

The level of violence of the escape is sometimes why you need the vomit rag. If you often get a milk shower and your partner does not, it may be that your feeding technique is encouraging the ingestion of air. It may be worthwhile to revisit your style and pay close attention to the differences between how you and your partner feed the baby. The little effort might save a few t-shirt changes.

Putting the Baby to Bed. Times where you may assume the greatest role as a hero is when you can manage to get the newborn asleep when your partner has been at it for hours. It is sometimes an achievement to develop confidence in getting them back to sleep in the middle of the night. Things that might keep a baby awake that are obvious to moms — and dads tend to forget — are a change of diapers or a bit of a nip at the baby bottle. Of course, gas of more than one sort may be keeping the baby awake with stomach or abdominal discomfort. A gentle massage may be just the thing.

Tricks do work sometimes, such as bringing the baby out for a ride in the stroller or the car. Cutting across a playing field once, I found that taking our stroller with super-sized wheels out over a lot of open grass created a motion that was lulling. The ride was a bit less smooth than the asphalt, and it seemed to be a trick that worked often. Be sure to keep car rides to those times you are alert enough to drive.

Another popular method to work with is sound. The womb environment is dark, and most of the fetus's sensory stimulation is auditory. Considering the baby is permanently submerged for those nine months, sounds tend to be muffled and rhythmic, like breathing or the pulsing of blood. So while people sometimes turn to what they recognize as music as something that will be lulling and comforting to a baby, it may not be the best choice. Lullabies were created for a reason, but sure, babies may prefer jazz, classical, new age, or even rock. When you find something that works, try and expand on that library. Don't be surprised if the sounds that lull your baby will not be those you find lulling yourself. It sounds like summer storms may have a similar effect on infants as they do on adults, and simple white noise like turning on the shower can be simple magic.

Pay attention to the position(s) your child prefers to fall asleep in, and if you never have, try different positions. Upright, cradled, and face down can all produce different results, as can rhythmic rocking or moving about with a bit of a bounce in your step.

Take care when placing the baby in the crib. The baby should always be placed on its back, especially in the early months when it cannot navigate on its own. Keep the immediate area free of plush toys, pillows, blankets, and other things that may look attractive to an adult but may not be best for the child's safety during sleep.

Parenting and Partnering Power

You have graduated from pregnancy school, and now you are a dad. The list of new skills you have to learn here is less mysterious when the pregnancy is over and the baby is here, mainly because you can see what you are working with. Pregnancy was fraught with emotions and the unknown processes you could not see, and in fatherhood, things are primarily hands-on and happen in the real world. That will be to your advantage. Take advice and learn from experience, and everything will be just fine.

Don't just chuck that daddy notebook. If luck should have it that you will be a parent to a newborn, later on, this will be a great record book of what happened. It will also be a way to learn about the mistakes you made because your personal record is going to be the most valuable thing you have going forward. Even if you have a good memory, that notebook will make it better.

Conclusion

A Sentimental Journey

You've seen the pregnancy through to completion successfully, and you have mostly managed not to botch anything. If you have given it your all, you have improved the state of your relationship, even if it was good before. You've enhanced what and how you share, which bodes well for the future.

The journey of pregnancy was one you took together and has unfolded in the blossoming of new life. If you have taken the advice in these pages seriously and followed up on suggestions, you had an easier time tackling this first experience with pregnancy than most men will, and you enhance the health and prospects of your relationship and family. This was not just a journey of sweat and tears; it was a learning experience that has made you a better partner and a better dad. Just like training for a job, the skills you learn will seep over into other parts of your life and help you embrace responsibilities you would never have trained for otherwise.

After the child is born, one distinct difference you may begin to notice between yourself and your partner is that she will tend to want these years to last forever. While you will have fun and enjoy the experience (most of the time), you might not be able to hold down your enthusiasm for getting your infant to do guy things with you, like playball. I admit that I wanted to start my first in games of skill a little too early. On the other hand, I did end up enjoying those years in a dad sort of way. I suggest that you don't rush these years of infancy. Just like you couldn't push the accelerator on the nine months of pregnancy, all will come in time. Prepare yourself to consider what else you can gain from this part of the experience. Some people call it mindlessness, living in the moment rather than constantly pushing toward the future or, worse, trying to change the past. If you waste the opportunity you have now, it won't come back. At some point, you may end up looking back with an empty portfolio of the early years of your child's life and wonder where they went.

It may be that you don't really have fun cooing and when a group of women get together to talk about babies, the whole sense of joy washes over you like words of gossip over a fence. You'll volunteer to fill snack bowls and top off drinks just to get out of the room. What you really want to do is look for those moments that end up being distinctly "dad." If cooing is not your thing, leave the cooing to mom and focus on the things in your child's world of wonder that you can enjoy. It isn't a good idea to go against your partner's wishes, but there are times I let my kids do things that might have made their mom frown. Nothing dumb like playing in kitty litter but exploring the world with not so nimble little fingers. When it came time to crawl around in the grass, being part of that experience by pointing out the dandelions and things that might ignite discovery created a different kind of joy. Showing a baby how to dunk an acorn into a plastic bucket is a skill level some will manage before their first words. But that is a connection and the beginning of communications with your kid. Things that became commonplace long ago to you are all new to your child's eyes, and maybe they are a way for you to see the world anew again. The smallest things might bring them the greatest satisfaction, and this tiny thing you brought into the world can, in turn, be that source of satisfaction and discovery for you.

I read to the children from a very young age, and all remain avid readers. My second child loved reading so much that she had a physical response to the words she read. It was like she was getting plugged in. One child walked so early she became a danger to herself, and I felt I had to follow her around like a human rubber baby bumper. Many times she'd end up heels overhead anyway. Another never crawled at all, instead of using her own creative means of locomotion (I've heard it called scooching and scooting). People would stare at her as she zipped down hallways in hotels cause she could really move. Each of them was like exploring a book uniquely about their discovery of the world and themselves. As they got older, I knew them better because I watched them develop, and their behavior arose as hints to what would make them uniquely themselves. I learned from them, and I hope they learned from me.

Soon enough, your kid will get to the age where you feel more in your element. You may even end up missing some of the more mundane things that came to pass as they grow because you can't be there all the time. But this whole process of mastering pregnancy and fatherhood is something no one is born with. It is a hard-fought battle of perseverance and will; still, the payoff is enormous. Learn to enjoy the moments, and they will stay with you forever.

Parenting and Partnering Power

You now have the tools to help you understand what is to come. My hope is you can now look forward to exploring the world that is opening up before you. Be a participant who is willing to learn and continue to grow by staying the course. This part of the journey means learning new things whilst relishing the memories. Dwell on the good ones. They say having a memory is virtually the same as living through the event. Pick and choose the good ones, and you are just adding scoops of the good ice cream on top of the cone.

I would be glad to hear your feedback about this book, both from the perspective of how it applied to your experience and what you learned from your real-life experience that could have been included here. Feel free to email me at: http://williamhardingauthor.com/.

If you think the book was helpful and that it is worthy of a nice review, please leave one on Amazon or your venue of choice. This will help dads that you don't even know to prepare for this phase of their life and look forward to enjoying their future.

Thanks for reading this work. I look forward to creating more in the future.

You may not be ready to do it again just yet, and your partner may not be either, but like everything that slides into the rear-view mirror of life, you can always look back with a greater appreciation.

Reviews

As an independent author with a small marketing budget, reviews are my livelihood on this platform. If you enjoyed this book, I'd really appreciate it if you left your honest feedback. I love hearing from my readers, and I personally read every single review.

Join The Dads Club Commuinty

DAD's Club: Support Group For Dads | Facebook

References

Is Couvade Syndrome (Sympathetic Pregnancy) Real? (healthline.com)

60 Great Quotes And Sayings On Fatherhood (firstcry.com)

Apgar score - Wikipedia

Made in United States
Orlàndo, FL
12 November 2022

24428666R00064